Successful and Sustainable Weight Loss

Uwe Knop

Successful and Sustainable Weight Loss

Evidence-Based Strategies to Slim Down and Maintain It

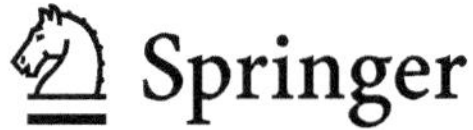
Springer

Uwe Knop
Echzell, Germany

ISBN 978-3-662-72476-7 ISBN 978-3-662-72477-4 (eBook)
https://doi.org/10.1007/978-3-662-72477-4

Translation from the German language edition: "Erfolgreich abnehmen und schlank bleiben" by Uwe Knop, © Der/die Herausgeber bzw. der/die Autor(en), exklusiv lizenziert an Springer-Verlag GmbH, DE, ein Teil von Springer Nature 2025. Published by Springer Berlin Heidelberg. All Rights Reserved.

This book is a translation of the original German edition "Erfolgreich abnehmen und schlank bleiben," 2nd edition, by Uwe Knop, published by Springer-Verlag GmbH, DE in 2025. The translation was done with the help of an artificial intelligence machine translation tool. A subsequent human revision was done primarily in terms of content, so that the book will read stylistically differently from a conventional translation. Springer Nature works continuously to further the development of tools for the production of books and on the related technologies to support the authors.

This Springer imprint is published by the registered company Springer-Verlag GmbH, DE, part of Springer Nature.
The registered company address is: Heidelberger Platz 3, 14197 Berlin, Germany

Preface to the Second Edition

Take a moment to think back to the half-decade from 2021 to 2025—and you will quickly realize: in these five years, a lot has happened on our planet, in politics, technology, AI (artificial intelligence), global networks, and on many other levels; perhaps even in your own personal life? However, in one area of science, there have been neither major "revolutionary game-changing discoveries" nor groundbreaking changes in direction in recent years—not even noteworthy new developments. By this, I mean the "science of *natural* weight loss." And the fact that the state of knowledge in this field has remained unchanged is anything but negative—quite the opposite, in fact—because it shows: **We have reached the end of wisdom. We know how it works, how weight loss functions—in principle.** And that is extremely gratifying.

Already during the conception of the first edition of this book, after years of intensive analysis of all relevant publications, statements, and guidelines, it became clear to me: In the field of natural weight loss, we are entering a new era, marked by a clear paradigm shift, which can be described as follows: The individual is at the center—not the weight loss model or even specific diet plans imposed on people. Even then, it was becoming increasingly evident that weight reduction programs have only a *chance* of being successful if they fulfill the following indispensable foundation:

Losing weight is always an entirely individual process—and this path to your desired weight must therefore always and exclusively be tailored to your own personality; it must fit perfectly with your unique lifestyle as well as your personal preferences and dislikes.

The era of "off-the-shelf classic diets" was already over back then—and it is even more so today. For what was a relatively new approach before 2021 has, by 2025, become the scientific standard. By now, it is likely that no professional society, no guideline, and no reputable scientist holds a different view: **Sustainable and successful weight reduction is only possible if the model fits the person—and not the other way around.**

Therefore, the past years have confirmed this book's pioneering role as a "foundational work on weight loss" at all levels—and thus, at its core, nothing fundamental has changed in the content: **The personal path to your desired weight has remained fundamentally the same.**

But: In the meantime, there have also been new studies, guidelines, and statements that impressively underscore the tenor of this book—and which are now an integral part of the essential knowledge conveyed in this new edition. And even though there have been no groundbreaking changes in the field of *natural* weight reduction, and the only truly effective approach has continued to establish itself consistently (which is great!)—there have, however, been significant developments in the area of pharmaceutical options: The now widely known "weight loss injections" are considered the revolutionary game changer for weight reduction. Therefore, in this new edition, you will also learn about the key opportunities and risks of these new "revolutionary slimming aids from the pharmaceutical lab"—and especially whether the expensive injections are worthwhile not only for the pharmaceutical companies, but also for the users… In addition, I have expanded the book with some very practical everyday tips that make the individual journey to your desired weight a bit easier.

In this spirit, I wish you every success in losing weight even more easily—and keeping it off—after reading the new edition!

Culinary regards, yours
nutritional scientist, Uwe Knop

Preface to the First Edition

Adele. The weight loss queen of 2020 is clearly singer Adele. With her ever-fresh slim-down snapshots, she delights her fans on social media. "She did it! Sensational!" The once curvy, Rubenesque singer with the powerhouse "Hello" voice reportedly lost a whopping 45 kg—rumor has it that she shed nearly half her body weight through a 1,000 kcal-per-day diet and intense training. Fans and followers were, and still are, absolutely thrilled—for her first bikini photo showcasing her new slim silhouette, she received a true wave of warm praise on Instagram in August 2020. "So great," "Amazing how you did it," "You look fantastic," "Cool new look, keep it up!" World stars aren't the only ones to experience this—those of us "regular people" who have lost a significant amount of weight for all to see are also familiar with these positive reactions, the affirmations, and the virtual pats on the back for a "superb" weight loss achievement. That's how it is these days: those who lose weight are celebrated. Slim is the new healthy, the new fit, the epitome of self-control, discipline, and mastery. The underlying message is: "I have myself and my life under control." Being slim is considered beautiful. You don't have to like it, but that's the reality. The times we live in, the reality of this era, must be accepted as they are—and for that reason, we should have full understanding for all women and men who want to lose weight. And there are many. Representative surveys consistently show similar results: in 2018, 71% of German women aged 16 to 44 wanted to lose weight (appinio 2018). In 2019, it was still about two-thirds (62%) (Pelikan 2019). Among men, nearly half said they wanted to reduce their weight (appinio 2018). Beyond the good feeling of "lightness," successful weight loss also sends a clear message to our achievement-oriented society: "I want it too, I can do it, and I feel good about it!" And that is exactly what this book provides: understanding for a wish that deserves to be fulfilled. Understanding for a goal that absolutely wants to be achieved: to become (and stay) slimmer. But this book offers not only understanding, but also the knowledge and tools you need to reach your goal. That is exactly where I want to support you, with all my expertise and knowledge as an evidence-focused graduate ecotrophologist, committed to science and comprehensive education.

For more than 14 years, I have been analyzing nutrition studies—now well over 6,000 publications—and interpreting the data free from ideologies, personal preferences, or economic interests, guided solely by truth, evidence, and my conscience. In my publications, lectures, and media interviews, diets have not fared well so far. For good scientific reason: because the evidence on diets unmistakably reveals that they are not effective in the long term and therefore do not lead to lasting weight loss.

If you want to lose weight, you need to know *everything*

So why is it that a nutrition scientist, who is familiar with the data and critically evaluates diets, is now writing a book about losing weight instead of a book warning against diets? The answer is actually quite simple: because many of us, especially women, want to diet. Not for the sake of dieting itself, but because the desire to lose weight, to become thinner, to be slim, ranks very high on most women's "life wish list." The reasons for this are varied and depend on the era: currently, there is a prevailing beauty ideal that not only preaches, propagates—and demands—a slim silhouette as the goal. Society also expects a fat-free, well-toned, muscular body that must be sculpted and revered—and it is by this standard that people in the Western world are measured. Being slim is equated with being healthy, attractive, and high-performing—whereas being overweight is nowadays associated with negative attributes such as lazy, unattractive, unhealthy, and weak. This creates pressure, which especially affects women, as their public presence and social role are judged even more strictly by the ideal of being slim, attractive, and fat-free than is the case for men. To make matters worse, with the omnipresent abundance of food and the often limited physical activity in office jobs, it is simply difficult for the many "sedentary knowledge workers" to remain effortlessly slim in the long term. As we age, it also becomes increasingly difficult, due to metabolic changes, to maintain a slim weight—women in menopause are particularly familiar with this phenomenon… And not just in themselves, because, take a moment to reflect: how many friends and acquaintances do you have who watch their figure, who repeatedly "want to lose a few kilos (or sometimes more)," who embark on a "spring diet" every year? Surely not a few, since both women and men often struggle with their body shape. "A little less fat, a few clothing sizes smaller, and some nicely toned muscles—that's something I would really like…"

So people go on diets, enroll in courses, buy books, book online seminars and coaching sessions, and "follow" social media slimming fitness influencers. On Facebook and Instagram, "slimming successes," thigh gaps, and ab cracks are posted, shared, and liked. Diets are a multi-billion dollar industry. Every year, new trendy diets hit the market, promising the dream body—especially when celebrities visibly slim down. For example, in mid-2020, the Sirtfood diet was on everyone's lips after media reports claimed that former soul singer Adele had—according to the familiar narrative—lost an incredible 45 kg with it. However, this is neither proven nor is the Sirtfood diet the new "super diet" that makes everyone slim. By the way: Adele could just as well have done a street food diet instead of Sirtfood—because her kilos didn't disappear because of *what* she ate, but because of what she *didn't* eat. That's why there are as many diets as there are grains of sand on the beach:

estimates suggest there are more than 500 different slimming variants. The mechanisms behind them are always the same. The potential risks and negative effects are also the same. All of this is well known, and the scientific community is in agreement. But: None of the diet providers have communicated this openly and honestly to date. Because: You have to stay "unique," that is, be one of a kind, in order to position the new slimming offer as marketable. Because, as so often, it's all about the money.

Many women and men want to lose weight, that is also a fact. And they go on these diets.

In the process, those wishing to lose weight are usually deceived with false promises: "Now, at last, there is finally the one diet that will truly make you slim forever." Every year, the diet fairy tale returns. Hopes are raised that, due to their unsuccessful dieting histories, drive many people struggling with their weight ever deeper into despair. And that is exactly what must stop!

So I decided to write this somewhat different book on sustainable weight loss, so that you, as someone wishing to lose weight, are fully, objectively, and transparently informed about everything that is truly important to know. Because only with this 360° comprehensive insight can you decide at the end of this "reading journey": Will I take the path of long-term weight reduction—or will I choose a different route? If you want to become slim, by the end of this book you will know exactly how this goal can be achieved and what you need to pay attention to.

Overview

This calls for a book that honestly makes clear:

- Losing weight is possible—in principle, anyone can become slim
- Because: The biological mechanism is very simple and is always the same in all diets
- However, maintaining the reduced weight is the "real art" that only a few master: 80–90% of all diets fail

- Because to stay on the path to success (permanently slim), you need not only perseverance, but also knowledge of the "how"
- And: There are real risks—including "weight relapse" (yo-yo effect and more)

Yes, there are ways and means to achieve your slim, feel-good weight—and, above all, to maintain it. To do so, you need to understand the fundamental principle behind weight loss and be aware of the risks involved before, during, and especially after the process. And you will gain this knowledge—because I particularly want to protect women, who are under enormous pressure to be slim, as well as all men who wish to lose weight, from continually falling for the ever-new diet myths peddled by clever power sellers, thereby gradually ruining their health and their weight. My intention is by no means to say: "It's better not to lose weight!" The decision whether you want to reduce your weight is one that each person must make for themselves. I will help you understand the principle of weight loss, apply it individually in your life, and thus achieve your goal: to become slim—and stay that way.

This open and honest book on sustainable weight loss lives up to this approach—uncompromisingly clear, authentic, and scientifically based on the latest research. No false promises, just the plain truth. My goal is that after reading, you will feel confident that you never need to read another diet book—because after this, you will know everything you need to know. There is nothing more to say or write on the subject.

So every woman and every man knows exactly what they are getting into when they embark on the "path of weight reduction"—with all its pros and cons. But then the motto should be: I DIET MY WAY. You follow your own, very personal path. Why? You will find out as you read.

But this path may not be an easy one, although you will feel lighter and relieved afterward. In this book, we begin your "journey to a new, slimmer you" by first dispelling diet myths. We then move on to self-reflection, self-awareness, and mindset. This is followed by the practical section, where you can discover and create your own personal, sustainable approach to nutrition and lifestyle change—one that fits you, your life and daily routine, your character and personality, and your goals. Last but not least, the book also offers an alternative, intuitive path to achieving your feel-good weight. In the end, you decide which path is right for you.

Enough of the preface—I wish you a wonderful "journey of discovery" toward your desired dream figure!

Spring 2021

Culinary regards, yours
nutritional scientist, Uwe Knop

Sources

appinio (2018) Diet Study: 71% of women currently want to lose weight. https://www.appinio.com/de/blog/di%C3%A4t-trend-ern%C3%A4hrung-fitness. Accessed 21. Feb. 2021

Pelikan M (2019) https://www.presseportal.de/pm/6788/4155679. Two out of three women want to lose weight. Accessed 21. Feb. 2021

Contents

About the Author

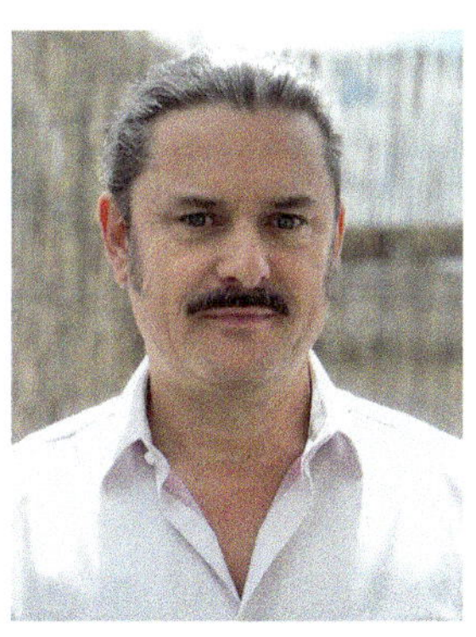

Uwe Knop (*72) is an evidence-focused nutrition scientist (Dipl.oec. troph./JLU Giessen), publicist, and author from the heart of Hesse. For more than 15 years, he has been analyzing current nutrition studies and has made it his goal to process the knowledge contained therein independently and free from third-party interests, and to present it in an understandable way. He believes that everyone should be able to inform themselves comprehensively and make conscious decisions, and ideally listen to themselves and their own bodies rather than to "external" advice of any kind. His sole intention is to encourage people to place greater trust in their intuitive body navigator and its guiding feelings of hunger, desire, satiety, and above all, tolerance.

Author for Burda/Focus online

Uwe Knop is a guest editorial author as a Focus Online expert and analyzes current studies and media reports here. You can access his author profile on Focus Online via the following link or QR code: https://www.focus.de/intern/impressum/autoren/uwe-knop_id_7576221.html

Speaker, Lecturer; Lectures & Presentations

In addition to his work as an author, Dipl.oec.troph. Knop also gives lectures and keynotes as a speaker, for example at professional associations, companies, and medical education events. Request a customized lecture on your desired nutrition topic at: uwe.knop@gmail.com

Book Publications

2021/2025—Successful weight loss and staying slim: Sustainable weight reduction scientifically proven (Springer-Verlag)

2024—FINALLY EATING RIGHT: Enjoy honestly with a clear conscience—Trust your ETHICS & INTUITION (KDP/Kindle-Direct-Publishing)

2020—Intuitive Intermittent Fasting (Polarise-Verlag)

2019—Your Body Navigator to the Best Food of All Time (Polarise-Verlag)

2017—Intuitive Eating (MVG/riva Publishing)

2017—Good Carbs: Why You Don't Need to Fear Bread and Pasta (MVG/riva-Verlag)

2017—Child, eat something (that you like!) (Plassen-Verlag)

2016—Nutrition Mania: Why We Don't Need to Be Afraid of Eating (Rowohlt-Verlag)

2009—Hunger & Lust: The first book on culinary body intelligence (BoD-Verlag)

1
All Diets Work the Same—But Some Work More Equally

The title of this chapter is freely adapted from the famous quote in George Orwell's Animal Farm: "All animals are equal. But some animals are more equal than others." Although this literary classic has little to do with diets, the statement fits perfectly, because: All diets work the same, as they operate on the same principle. However, providers position their diets as different, as "more equal," as better than all the others. In reality, there are no relevant differences. You will learn why this is the case on the following pages.

> At the center of this is the "revelation" of the human-biologically universal weight loss principle of all diets: the negative energy balance. This means: taking in less energy than you expend. During this hypocaloric (i.e., energy-deficient) phase, our body must use up its own energy stores (fat, muscle), and we lose mass and weight.

Let's start with a brief excursion into the paradoxical business practices of the diet industry—because you should be aware of the main pitfalls of the various diet providers before we then turn specifically to the two

U. Knop, *Successful and Sustainable Weight Loss*,
https://doi.org/10.1007/978-3-662-72477-4_1

probably most popular "slimming hypes of modern times"—and then get to the core of the book.

Let's begin the chapter with a fairly recent diet study in the *Journal of Clinical Lipodology* (Porter Starr et al. 2019): Researchers at the Duke University School of Medicine (USA) were actually able to show that a calorie-reduced diet, in which lean red meat provided the (slightly increased) protein intake, led to significant weight loss in the participants. And that's not all: The results also suggested that this hypocaloric diet (= too little energy), with either traditional (0.8 g per kg body weight per day) or higher protein content (1.2 g per kg body weight per day), consumed mainly as lean red meat, improved risk markers for cardiovascular disease and type II diabetes in obese middle-aged and older adults. Both diets were also associated with improved physical function and showed no adverse effects on cardiometabolic events. Great, all the steak aficionados rejoice, "There it is: the first red meat diet that makes you slim and healthy!" But let's not get carried away—because this study, too, shows only one thing: how arbitrary diets are.

1.1 Diets—A Gateway Drug to ...

People who have already been through several diets know from lived experience: diets do not make you slim, but rather make you gain weight in the long run. This is because weight-loss regimens cause our bodies to switch their energy balance to low power, and after the diet, the lost kilos are regained—with an added safety margin to be prepared for the next "famine." This is the well-known yo-yo effect. The rule is: the more diets, the longer the dieting career, the more pronounced the "kilo relapse."

"The more often you subject your body to such periods of hunger, the more you gain afterwards, because the body does not know you are fasting intentionally, and stores up energy reserves out of fear of these (seemingly recurring) 'famines.'" (Schumacher 2021)

These findings are no longer a conspiratorial secret, but rather scientific consensus that is repeatedly emphasized in public.

As early as the end of 2012, a survey by the Society for Consumer Research GfK (Kolb 2012) confirmed what science knows but the diet industry prefers to conceal: 73 percent of women experienced with dieting were either heavier or just as heavy one year after the diet as before the starvation cure. This representative survey of women supports the findings of numerous international and German scientists. For example, the two Swiss nutrition scientists Dulloo and Montani from the University of Fribourg (Bartens 2016) stated: "After at most one year, you have regained one to two thirds of the weight originally lost, and after five years, the rest." One third of people who try to lose weight are hit especially hard: they end up weighing even more than at the start of their diet. This matches the observation of the former president of the German Nutrition Society (DGE), Prof. Helmut Heseker: "We know that 80 to 90 percent of all weight reduction programs are unsuccessful." On the contrary: "Often, participants end up even heavier than before," Heseker explained as early as the beginning of 2012 to the *Welt* (Kunz 2012). And his colleague Prof. Andreas Pfeiffer from Charité in Berlin and the German Institute of Human Nutrition (DIfE) confirms this finding (Preuk 2013): "90 percent gain weight again after the end of the diet."

Even more alarming results were provided by a large review study in the *American Journal of Public Health* (Fildes et al. 2015): The researchers analyzed data from 77,000 obese women and 100,000 obese men who tried to lose weight through various weight-loss programs. A few years after the diet, the success rate looked more than meager:

> Only 0.8 percent of women reached normal weight; among men, the rate was even lower, at less than half a percent (0.47 percent). These authors also conclude that common weight-loss programs and diets are ineffective.

In this context, the clarifications by researchers in a "Scientific Statement" in the journal *Endocrine Reviews* (Schwarz et al. 2017) on the development of obesity are interesting: "Body weight reduced by diets—lower than the biologically defended level—leads to increased hunger and creates the perfect metabolic storm for the body to regain its biologically preferred weight. This should be expected by both patients and physicians as a physically normal response to dieting."

Therefore: Whether intermittent fasting, Atkins, Slim in Your Sleep, Paleo, Low Carb, Keto, Vegan, Sirtfood, or any of the other 478 diets—one thing applies to all trends:

> No diet makes you slim in the long term, because hardly anyone can stick to a reduced-calorie diet for life. After the diet, people return to normal eating and their original weight comes back—usually with a "safety margin" for future "famines."

But former dieters not only become heavier again, but usually also fatter—because during the diet, the body also breaks down muscle mass, while during the yo-yo weight regain, mostly only fat is stored. According to a study in the top journal *Lancet* (Purcell et al. 2014), it does not matter whether you lost weight slowly over 36 weeks or shed the same number of kilos in twelve turbo weeks. The majority of the weight comes back to all former dieters with a "fat safety margin," as a subsequent review from the University of Montreal (Atallah et al. 2014) showed, which compared Atkins, South Beach, Weight Watchers, and other commercial diets. The modest weight loss in the diet year was comparable, but after two years, study participants weighed either the same as before or even more. The conclusion of numerous other review studies in medical journals confirms these findings:

> Whether low-carb, low-fat, or high-protein—diets do not help with long-term weight loss.

As early as 2013, the German Institute for Medical Documentation and Information (DIMDI), an institute within the portfolio of the Federal Ministry of Health (BMG), published a more than 150-page report on the "Effectiveness of Diets for Sustainable Weight Reduction in Overweight and Obesity" (Korczak and Kister 2013). The researchers analyzed exclusively 33 diet studies of the highest possible quality—and their conclusion is clear: "Overall, the study results show that all diets tested are effective …

… there is no evidence that any specific diet is superior to all others …

… that is, moderately fat-reduced, calorie-reduced, protein- or carbohydrate-rich diets achieve nearly the same effect. The effectiveness of a vegan diet for weight stabilization appears to be weaker, as does that of meal replacement or formula diets" (Korczak and Kister 2013).

Numerous subsequent studies have repeatedly reproduced and confirmed this "universal finding of non-superiority." This is also true for one of the most recent and largest reviews, published in February 2020 in the renowned medical journal *BMJ British Medical Journal* (Ge et al. 2020):

All diets are comparably effective—but only in the short term.

This sobering but expected finding was reached by the Canadian researchers after analyzing data from more than 21,000 overweight individuals from 121 studies who participated in 14 different scientifically supervised diet programs. The meta-analysis included both low-carb and low-fat diets as well as branded programs like Weight Watchers, South Beach, or DASH. After half a year, the majority of participants had lost about the same amount of weight, around 4–5 kg—regardless of which of the 14 diets they had followed, it made no difference. The proportion of meat or vegetables in the respective diet also had no effect on weight loss. In general, their overall health improved slightly, as shown by various cardiovascular laboratory parameters such as blood pressure. But already one year after the diet, the positive effects had almost disappeared. In line with this:

"If diets worked in the long term, there wouldn't constantly be new ones." (ÖKOTEST 2021)

1.2 The Type of Diet Does Not Matter

Because at the end of the study, twelve months later, many had regained weight. On average, they weighed only 2 kg less compared to their starting weight. The study leaders clearly state that even at the 12-month endpoint, it is in fact irrelevant which of the different diets participants used for weight reduction, because: differences between the diets were hardly detectable even at the end. The authors' conclusion is therefore unequivocally clear: Basically, it does not matter which diet is chosen for weight loss, because: they are all very similar. However:

What is crucial, however, is to stick with the diet in the long term. People should therefore choose the diet that appeals to them most, the one that best suits them and their individual lifestyle.

1.3 Thousands of Diets—One Principle of Action

This common knowledge is understandable, because—as already indicated at the outset—the fact is: All diets work according to the same principle: a negative energy balance, meaning consuming fewer calories than are expended. This forces the body to tap into its reserves in order to maintain its metabolism. Numerous scientists repeatedly emphasize that the type of diet is completely irrelevant. And this was already clarified in 2014 by the German Obesity Society in its guidelines (Berg et al. 2014):

"In a diet, the composition of carbohydrates, fat, and protein plays hardly any role; the only thing that matters is the total calorie count." How the energy deficit is achieved is irrelevant.

A comparable conclusion was reached shortly thereafter by one of the largest analyses to date, published in the world-renowned medical journal *JAMA* (Johnston et al. 2014): The evaluation of about 50 studies found no difference between different types of diets. The negative energy balance is thus the secret behind even the most mysterious diet. This means, conversely: The wonderful-sounding stories surrounding the various trendy diets are nothing more than made-up tales to boost sales. "Feast for 5 days, fast for 2," "no carbs in the evening," "eat vegan," "inject HCG hormones," "do gene and blood tests"—no matter what is served up to women wanting to lose weight (almost 90 percent of dieters are female): Every year, the new trendy diet plays with the hopes of many disappointed women and men who have already tried countless diets—always without success.

1.4 Failure as a Business Model

The fact is: There is no diet that makes you slim permanently. And this is understandable, because otherwise there wouldn't be a new diet hype every year. This, in turn, pleases the diet industry, incidentally the only economic sector that generates billions because its products do not work; because they do not deliver what they promise. But it is precisely with this paradoxical business model that the slimming industry maintains its—in both senses—growing target group. "If the product worked, there would be no business to be made from it," revealed the former financial director of Weight Watchers in the BBC documentary "The Slimmers" from 2014. In this remarkable two-part TV documentary, other diet providers are also interviewed, who candidly admit: Of course, losing weight doesn't work that easily, but that's exactly what's so great about it—from their perspective.

1.5 Genes and Hunger Hormones Prevent Us from Losing Weight

The cause for this lies, incidentally, in our genetic makeup: Research suggests that our body weight is determined 70–80 percent by our genes. Accordingly, US researchers from the Columbia University Medical Center in New York announced in a *Lancet* study (Ochner et al. 2015): Obesity is not to be treated with dietary calorie reduction, because the body's biology subsequently restores its natural weight.

In 2018, researchers at the Norwegian University of Science and Technology confirmed in their publication in the *American Journal of Physiology, Endocrinology and Metabolism* (Coutinho et al. 2017): A central regulator of the yo-yo effect is that after successful forced weight reduction, the body increases secretion of the hunger hormone "ghrelin." The subjects' feelings of hunger were significantly stronger both one and even two years after the diet than at the beginning.

Conclusion of the researchers: Anyone who loses a significant amount of weight must expect increased feelings of hunger for years. And most likely, this will persist until the genetic makeup (the genes) have restored the body's "original weight."

This is echoed by Prof. Matthias Blüher, head of the Obesity Outpatient Clinic for Adults at Leipzig University Medicine and president of the German Obesity Society, who clarified the question "Are overweight and obese people themselves to blame for their excess weight?" on the independent diabetes portal diabsite.de (Blüher 2018): "No, that's not true. We now know, for example, that genetic factors play a very large role in the development of overweight and obesity. Hormonal aspects and our social environment also contribute to the development of overweight. None of these factors can be actively influenced by the individual."

Blüher further clarified (Wesely 2018): "In addition, our body tries to maintain its highest achieved weight. It defends it vehemently …

This means for the body to lower its basal metabolic rate and energy expenditure so much that it can defend its weight even with little food ..." Furthermore, the obesity expert regretted that, unfortunately, one must say that weight loss concepts based solely on eating less and moving more have failed in the long term, because the body defends its starting weight again. Specifically, his experience is as follows: "Some of my patients diet and gain weight in the process. This weight gain is not yet understood scientifically. We cannot explain it. How the body utilizes the calories consumed and regulates the basal metabolic rate cannot be consciously controlled by humans."

Diets are a trap that snaps shut in several ways: For most people, they do not make them slimmer, but rather make them fatter in the long run, so that they fall into a vicious cycle and keep trying new diets. In the process, those wanting to lose weight often lose quite a bit of money on books, special foods, slimming powders, course fees, and more. And that's not all ...

1.6 Obesity and Eating Disorders

Diets are considered a "gateway drug" to obesity and eating disorders. Why is that? One reason is that many women and men become increasingly overweight due to the yo-yo effect. Due to higher social beauty pressures, the constant battle against one's own bodily sensations and food cravings can especially lead to eating disorders in women.

> "Anyone who diets from time to time knows the disappointment: this up and down is also called the yo-yo effect. So far, not even the most revolutionary diet has managed to overcome it." (Schumacher 2021)

This negative spiral is intensified by the feeling of failure—you have lost the battle against your own body, you have to cope with a major defeat. And you have to admit this not only to yourself, but also publicly to your family, friends, and colleagues. None of this brings joy; instead, it fuels deep-seated frustration that can become chronic. Paradoxically, even weight loss success seems to have negative consequences, at least according to the results of a study by University College London (Jackson et al. 2014). Heavier people who have successfully lost weight suffer more frequently from depressive disorders (why this is so can only be speculated—as is often the case with correlations and the question of chicken and egg). Here, the electrifying diet invention from the University of Lübeck (Labahn 2014) would be a promising approach to kill two birds with one stone: Electrical stimulation of the brain through the skull (transcranial) "reduces appetite and food intake without any diet—and this non-invasive method is already being used as an adjunct in the treatment of psychiatric disorders."

All in all, based on the scientific findings described, the only recommendation can really be: Stay away from classic diets! A diet-free life could not only be good for mental and physical health, it also strengthens sexual and social relationships—at least if one is to believe more recent research, which holds quite a few surprises.

It should be noted that correlations, i.e., statistical associations, should be viewed with a healthy dose of skepticism (more on this in Chap. 16). Therefore, as you read the following research findings, focus on the smile and chuckle effect that the study results may elicit in you.

1.7 Sex, Aggression, and Infidelity

A British consumer survey found that (statistically speaking) for every three kilos lost, you lose a friend. The reason is said to be jealousy over the dieting success—fortunately, that doesn't last long. Hopefully, not only the kilos but also the friends will return. But it's not just among friends that things can get tense when the kilos drop; stress with one's own partner is also common: Ohio State University (dpa 2019) reported that hungry couples argue more aggressively (surely everyone who has ever had nerve-wracking conversations while extremely hungry can relate). And the University of Texas (Shipman 2013) warned that one partner's attempts to lose weight can endanger the relationship, as the "dieter" either tries to convert the partner or the partner sabotages the diet. Both are toxic to a harmonious relationship.

On the other hand, the so-called "cuddle hormone" oxytocin ensures that kissing and caressing couples eat less. Perhaps kissing helps avoid the general desire to diet, which in turn would benefit a happy relationship. According to some assumptions, women are more likely to have affairs during a diet (the lack of energy weakens willpower, making them more susceptible to men's advances). However, if a man and woman remain faithful and happily married, the likelihood increases that both will gain weight over the years. This effect, however, could be counteracted as long as the woman remains fertile, because according to research from the Max Planck Institute (Braun 2013), fertility can help keep you slim. Perhaps couples should focus more on reproduction, since sex not only makes you happy but also burns calories—some men burn more calories during sex than during sports.

1.8 Brown Fat, Good Fat

Brown fat? These are the "good" fat layers that literally turn excess energy into hot air and are therefore in the research spotlight as "weight loss helpers." The more of these cells a person has, the more dietary energy can simply be burned as heat instead of ending up on the hips. There are numerous recent research findings on this, as scientists see a promising new "therapy target" here: "Brown fat cells for weight loss. Scientists from the Max Planck Institute for Metabolism Research in Cologne, the Medical University of Vienna, and the University of Southern Denmark in Odense are researching the function and regulation of brown fat cells, as these burn a lot of calories and are therefore ideally suited as the body's own cells for therapeutic options for weight reduction. Activating brown fat cells represents a novel way to lose weight," according to the optimistic tone of a press release (Burkert 2018). Researchers at the Medical University of Vienna agreed (Kiefer 2020), announcing in their study: Those who have brown fat burn about 15 percent more calories—but only if the "brown fat subjects" were briefly exposed to moderate cold. And that was not all the Viennese scientists were able to show: People with active brown fat tissue also had more anti-inflammatory fatty acids in their bodies, while simultaneously having lower concentrations of harmful fatty acids associated with diabetes or heart disease. "This shows us that we need to study human brown fat more closely to see whether activating this organ can protect us from metabolic and cardiovascular diseases," explained the study leader, Prof. Florian W. Kiefer from the Department of Internal Medicine III at the Medical University of Vienna. And that's not all: "Non-shivering thermogenesis [heat production] is the mechanism typical of brown fat for generating heat, but it not only consumes energy. The studies reveal that non-shivering thermogenesis is also a prerequisite for the feeling of satiety to occur in the brain," explained researchers at the Technical University of Munich (Klingenspor 2018) on the occasion of their new publication.

1.9 Moving in Together—Gaining Weight Together

In addition to sex, brown fat, and various other factors, the research collaboration between the Max Planck Institute for Human Development, the University of Mannheim, the University of Leipzig, and the German Institute for Economic Research (Skork 2018) published the following study results: "Couples have a higher body weight than singles—regardless of whether they are married or not. Contrary to previous assumptions, it is not so much marriage itself but rather moving in together for the first time that leads to weight gain." Thus, couples gain about twice as much weight after moving in together as couples do in the first four years of marriage. For the researchers, this means: This weight gain is primarily related to the change in relationship status. "A change in relationship status often also means a change in everyday eating habits—for example, having breakfast together, which might not have happened alone or would have been more modest." They suspect that food simply tastes better in company and that people generally eat more and thus consume more calories. If couples separate, the body mass index of both women and men generally drops back to the level it was before moving in together.

1.10 Stool Versus Kilos

So, to conclude this chapter, let's turn to an interesting "special diet from the intestinal depths." The fact that the composition of the approximately 100 trillion bacteria in the gut (formerly "gut flora," now: microbiota or microbiome) is related to our body weight is now undisputed. In short: Microbiome A lives mainly in the intestines of slim people, bacterial population B thrives in the guts of heavier people. Now, guess what idea researchers came up with?

The gut microbes of the slim are transferred to overweight patients via stool transplantation, and then the millions of little helpers assist with weight loss all on their own. "Foreign stool makes you slim," headlined the *Ärzte-Zeitung* (EB 2013) in an article about a Washington University study that made mice deliberately fat or slim via fecal transfer. A little later, the German Society for Mucosal Immunology and Microbiome e. V. (Mannsdorfer 2014) concluded: "It is obvious that stool transplantation, which has recently come increasingly into the focus of scientists, could be a new option in obesity therapy." However, it does take some getting used to: In their study at Ben-Gurion University of the Negev in Israel (Rinott et al. 2020), researchers showed that taking microbiome capsules made from one's own processed stool can counteract renewed weight gain. So you swallow your own… okay, let's stop here before anyone's imagination leads them to vomit on this lovely book.

1.11 Is Obesity Actually Contagious?

Scientists from the "Humans and the Microbiome" program at the Canadian Institute for Advanced Research (CIFAR), with participation from the Christian-Albrechts-University of Kiel (Pawlowski

2020), launched another rather bold approach regarding the microbiome: "Obesity, heart disease, or diabetes could be transmissible." The research team provided evidence that many diseases previously classified as non-communicable may in fact be passed from person to person via the microbiome. "If our revolutionary hypothesis proves correct, it will completely redefine our understanding of public health," explains Brett Finlay, professor of microbiology at the University of British Columbia and head of the CIFAR research program. What would be the consequences? Just imagine the hysteria if getting too close to an overweight person could "infect" you with obesity! And, humorously, on a first date: Man and woman want to be sure: "Have you been tested for fattening bacteria?" "Yes, and unfortunately I'm infected…" "Waiter, the bill please!"

1.12 Microbiome Analysis: Expensive and Ineffective

To avoid the aforementioned "date scenario," curious individuals have their stool analyzed for bacterial diversity: this is called microbiome analysis, which is not cheap. But does it actually help? In this context, the clear position of the German Society for Gastroenterology, Digestive and Metabolic Diseases (DGVS) (Pfeiffer 2018) is to be welcomed: Gastroenterology specialists unequivocally advise against using stool tests to examine the microbiome. These currently lack a scientific basis. "Microbiome research is still relatively in its infancy: which correlations exist and how they affect individuals is not yet sufficiently understood. Furthermore, the analytics do not yet provide consistent results that would be comparable between different laboratories," explains Prof. Stefan Schreiber, Director of the Department of Internal Medicine I at Kiel University Hospital. Nevertheless, some manufacturers and laboratories offer stool sample analyses for "analysis" of the gut flora and derive dietary and behavioral recommendations from the results. Regarding these stool tests for analyzing the gut microbiome, the medical experts of the DGVS professional society have a clear opinion: "Expensive and pointless!"

If, while reading the previous lines "from the depths of the charming gut," you are experiencing a mix of emotions—disbelief, amusement, and disgust—don't worry, we are almost at the end of the chapter, which calls for a clear mind and clear words, which two experts will now serve up for you …

1.13 ARD Exposes Diet Myths

In a highly recommended ARD documentary (Schickling 2020) on diet myths, there were clear statements that you should also be aware of. For example, Prof. Andreas Fritsche, who researches at the Chair of Nutritional Medicine and Prevention at the University Hospital Tübingen, explained why diets are so hard to stick to:

"When we lose weight, it is an emergency signal for the body. Our metabolism and genes actually come from the jungle, where food was scarce; this is deeply embedded in our metabolic programming, and the body then does everything it can to prevent weight loss. It lowers the basal metabolic rate and tries to regain weight—and that usually prevents weight loss."

And his research colleague Prof. Christine Brombach, Zurich University of Applied Sciences, answered the crucial question in the same report (Schickling 2020): "But when people have lost weight, can they manage to keep the reduced weight off?":

"If, right after the period of fasting, that is, losing weight, the diet, I don't really change my eating habits, then I simply fall into this yo-yo effect. That means I have a permanent reduction in my metabolism, and the studies are not entirely clear as to whether, by doing such a diet, I am not permanently setting my metabolism to a lower level and thus actually need less energy in the long term—and then, in the future, I constantly have to pay attention to how much total energy I consume, so as not to end up with more kilos on my back than before."

But if all diets work equally well in the short term, why is it so hard for us to stay slim in the long run? Because we know from numerous studies that most people weigh more after a diet than before—the infamous yo-yo effect …

Brombach adds: "The recommendation is that you should lose a maximum of about one kilo of body weight per week. Quite simply, to avoid crashing into this yo-yo effect. If you lose significantly more in a relatively short time under a strict regime, it is often this deceptive success because you have lost a lot of water. This rapid weight loss with water actually achieves nothing, and in the end, I have a less favorable body composition than before—in other words, if I lose weight too quickly, I actually have a much worse starting position than before the diet." (Schickling 2020)

The editorial team summarized as follows: Diet providers always sell a particular system, but basically, they are all crutches to help me eat less in some way?

The conclusion is: "Yes, you could put it that way; in the end, it's also a question of the energy I take in and the energy I expend" (Schickling 2020). The negative calorie balance says it all … Also interesting: In addition to reduced energy intake, many diets involve a strict schedule for meal times. Does that really make a difference? Does the time of eating really matter?

Once again, Professor Brombach: "It must be said quite simply: Ultimately, what matters is the total energy I consume over the course of the day. It's not about eating less or nothing at all in the evening. That is not scientifically proven. If you decide to lose weight, it is more or less irrelevant whether you skip breakfast or dinner. For example, there is also intermittent fasting—in the long term, it must be said, this form of diet does not perform better than other forms of calorie reduction. There are also no studies proving that it makes sense to separate carbohydrates and proteins in the evening." (Schickling 2020)

The editorial team also looked at daily rations from various diet concepts. Each of these concepts promises particularly efficient success. For example, the Atkins diet: complete avoidance of carbohydrates. Or "Slim in Your Sleep": separating protein and carbohydrates in meals. Or formula diets, which replace entire meals with a protein shake. But from the perspective of the ARD TV experts, the same principle works in every diet, which you now know inside and out: the consistent reduction of calorie intake.

The Most Important Points of the Chapter

- Diets do not make you slim in the long term, but often make you gain more weight.
- Which diet you choose does not matter, because: All diets work in the short term according to the same principle: negative energy balance (consuming fewer calories than you burn).
- There is no diet that works equally well for everyone.
- Interesting side note: A publication in *JAMA* made it clear that "weight-focused public health interventions provide no benefit but do cause some harm," because:
  Although the goal of these interventions is to reduce obesity, the percentage of the targeted groups with increased BMI has continued to rise, and accordingly, so has the proportion of those suffering from weight stigma and body dissatisfaction (Richmond et al. 2020). What does this also tell us: General measures and impersonal off-the-shelf appeals to lose weight are ineffective.

1.14 Summary of Key Messages: Your Current State of Knowledge

Initial note: This page is the "red thread of knowledge"—your current state of knowledge—that weaves continuously through the book. After each chapter, you will read the key messages so far—supplemented by the new essences of the current chapter, which are visually highlighted in bold at the end.

At this point in your journey to your new desired weight, you now know …

- **All diets are based on the same principle: negative energy balance.**
- **There is no better or worse diet—all diets are the same.**
- **Most weight loss programs fail and lead to weight gain because they are both impersonal and not tailored to the individual, and are only carried out for a short period.**
- **The result: The vicious circle/circulus vitiosus:**
  (new) diet fails ➔ weight gain ➔ fear of failure/self-doubt ➔ (new) diet fails ➔ …
- **Classic diets are therefore considered a "gateway drug" to eating disorders and obesity.**

References

Atallah et al (2014) Long-term effects of 4 popular diets on weight loss and cardiovascular risk factors. Circulation. https://doi.org/10.1161/CIRCOUTCOMES.113.000723

Bartens W (2016) Jojo-Effekt nach Diät ist ein Gesundheitsrisiko. https://www.sueddeutsche.de/gesundheit/diaeten-jojo-mortale-1.3250645. Accessed: 3. Sept. 2020

Berg et al (2014) Interdisziplinäre Leitlinie der Qualität S3 zur „Prävention und Therapie der Adipositas". https://www.awmf.org/uploads/tx_szleitlinien/050-001l_S3_Adipositas_Pr%C3%A4vention_Therapie_2014-11-abgelaufen.pdf. Accessed: 3. Sept. 2020

Blüher M (2018) Sieben Ernährungsmythen aufgeklärt. https://www.diabsite.de/aktuelles/nachrichten/2018/180815.html. Accessed: 3. Sept. 2020

Braun T (2013) Fruchtbarkeit hält schlank. https://www.mpg.de/7465730/fruchtbarkeit_und_uebergewicht. Accessed: 3. Sept. 2020

Burkert A (2018) Braune Fettzellen zum Abnehmen. https://idw-online.de/de/news701722. Accessed: 3. Sept. 2020

Coutinho et al (2017) Impact of weight loss achieved through a multidisciplinary intervention on appetite in patients with severe obesity. Am J Physiol Endocrinol Metabol. https://doi.org/10.1152/ajpendo.00322.2017

dpa (2019) Hunger lässt Paare aggressiver werden. https://www.fr.de/wissen/hunger-laesst-paare-aggressiver-werden-11226025.html. Accessed: 3. Sept. 2020

EB (2013) Fremder Kot macht schlank. https://www.aerztezeitung.de/Medizin/Fremder-Kot-macht-schlank-268561.html. Accessed: 3. Sept. 2020

Fildes et al (2015) Probability of an obese person attaining normal body weight: cohort study using electronic health records. https://doi.org/10.2105/AJPH.2015.302773

Ge et al (2020) Comparison of dietary macronutrient patterns of 14 popular named dietary programmes for weight and cardiovascular risk factor reduction in adults: systematic review and network meta-analysis of randomised trials. BMJ 369. https://doi.org/10.1136/bmj.m696

Jackson et al (2014) Psychological changes following weight loss in overweight and obese adults: a prospective cohort study. https://doi.org/10.1371/journal.pone.0104552

Johnston et al (2014) Comparison of weight loss among named diet programs in overweight and obese adults: a meta-analysis. JAMA 312(9). https://doi.org/10.1001/jama.2014.10397

Kiefer F (2020) Neue Erkenntnisse zur Wirkung von „braunem Fett" beim Menschen. https://www.meduniwien.ac.at/web/ueber-uns/news/detailseite/2020/news-im-april-2020/neue-erkenntnisse-zur-wirkung-von-braunem-fett-beim-menschen/. Accessed: 3. Sept. 2020

Klingenspor M (2018) Wie der Darm mit dem Braunen Fett „spricht". https://www.tum.de/studium/studinews/ausgabe-012011/show-012011/article/35085/. Accessed: 3. Sept. 2020

Kolb A (2012) Gesellschaft für Konsumforschung, Thema: Diäten, September/Oktober 2012. https://www.echte-esser.de/tl_files/files/GfK_Umfrage_Uwe-Knop_Diaeten_12-10-09.pdf. Accessed: 3. Sept. 2020

Korczak, Kister (2013) Wirksamkeit von Diäten zur nachhaltigen Gewichtsreduktion bei Übergewicht und Adipositas. Schriftenreihe Health Technology Assessment, Bd 127. https://portal.dimdi.de/de/hta/hta_berichte/hta345_bericht_de.pdf. Accessed: 3. Sept. 2020

Kunz M (2012) Diät fängt im Kopf an. Welt am Sonntag. https://www.welt.de/print/wams/vermischtes/article13803669/Diaet-faengt-im-Kopf-an.html. Accessed: 3. Sept. 2020

Labahn R (2014) Elektrische Hirnstimulation reduziert Appetit und Nahrungsaufnahme ohne Diät. https://idw-online.de/en/news600848. Accessed: 3. Sept. 2020

Mannsdorfer K (2014) Mit Bakterien gegen Adipositas? http://dgmim.de/index.php?id=318undL=%271. Accessed: 03. Sept. 2020

Ochner et al (2015) Treating obesity seriously: when recommendations for lifestyle change confront biological adaptations. Lancet Diabetes Endocrinol. https://doi.org/10.1016/S2213-8587(15)00009-1

ÖKOTEST (2021) Richtig abnehmen: Was Diäten tatsächlich bringen – und was nicht. https://www.oekotest.de/gesundheit-medikamente/Richtig-abnehmen-Was-Diaeten-tatsaechlich-bringen%2D%2Dund-was-nicht_104098_1.html. Accessed: 10.01.2021

Pawlowski B (2020) Adipositas, Herzkrankheiten oder Diabetes könnten übertragbar sein. https://idw-online.de/de/news730190. Accessed: 3. Sept. 2020

Pfeiffer J (2018) Teuer und sinnlos: DGVS rät von Stuhltests zur Analyse des Darm-Mikrobioms ab. https://www.dgvs.de/wp-content/uploads/2018/09/PM_2018_09_Stuhltests-Mikrobiom.pdf. Accessed: 3. Sept. 2020

Porter Starr et al (2019) Impact on cardiometabolic risk of a weight loss intervention with higher protein from lean red meat: combined results of 2 randomized controlled trials in obese middle-aged and older adults. J Clin Lipodol. https://doi.org/10.1016/j.jacl.2019.09.012.

Preuk M (2013) Krank statt schlank – Die zehn schlechtesten Diäten. https://www.focus.de/gesundheit/ernaehrung/abnehmen/tid-20983/schlankheits-diaet-macht-dick-krank-statt-schlank-die-zehn-schlechtesten-diaeten_aid:589657.html. Accessed: 3. Sept. 2020

Purcell et al (2014) The effect of rate of weight loss on long-term weight management: a randomised controlled trial. Lancet. https://doi.org/10.1016/S2213-8587(14)70200-1

Richmond et al (2020) Weight-focused public health interventions – no benefit, some harm. JAMA Pediatr. https://doi.org/10.1001/jamapediatrics.2020.4777

Rinott et al (2020) Effects of diet-modulated autologous fecal microbiota transplantation on weight regain. Gastroenterology. https://doi.org/10.1053/j.gastro.2020.08.041

Schickling K (2020) Abnehmen und schlank bleiben – kann das gehen? https://www.ardmediathek.de/alpha/video/alpha-thema/abnehmen-und-schlank-bleiben-kann-das-gehen/ard-alpha/Y3JpZDovL2JyLmRlL3ZpZGVvLzE0ZmRlZDc5LWQzYjUtNDA4NC1hZmFkLTIyOTZiZDFmMDBiNg/. Accessed: 16.10.2020

Schumacher B (2021) Schlank ohne Jo-Jo-Effekt: Wie Sie Ihr Gewicht halten. https://www.oekotest.de/gesundheit-medikamente/Schlank-ohne-Jo-Jo-Effekt-Wie-Sie-Ihr-Gewicht-halten-_107323_1.html. Accessed: 10.01.2021

Schwarz et al (2017) Obesity pathogenesis: an endocrine society scientific statement. Endocr Rev 38(4):267–296. https://doi.org/10.1210/er.2017-00111

Shipman M (2013) Weight loss not always beneficial for romantic relationships. https://news.ncsu.edu/2013/10/wms-romo-weight-2013/. Accessed: 3. Sept. 2020

Skork K (2018) Das Gewicht der Liebe: Wer zusammenzieht, nimmt zu. https://www.mpib-berlin.mpg.de/pressemeldungen/das-gewicht-der-liebe?c=2537. Accessed: 3. Sept. 2020

Wesely S (2018) „Abnehmen kann man nur mit dem Kopf". https://www.saechsische.de/plus/abnehmen-kann-man-nur-mit-dem-kopf-5017442.html. Accessed: 3. Sept. 2020

2
Trend Diets: Low Carb and Intermittent Fasting

Even if all diets are equally (in)effective, as you know: some are more equal than others… and so there are always a few current "hype diets" that, for a time, dominate all others in terms of media presence and public attention. In 1977, for example, this was the Vogue Diet, which promised women a weight loss of 2.5 kg in three days—by consuming a whole bottle of white wine daily, black coffee, hard-boiled eggs, and a pepper steak in the evening. The suggestion to start this diet on the weekend seems quite understandable, given the generous wine component… ideas like this are (unfortunately?) no longer in vogue today.

Instead, since 2017, two types of diets have consistently topped the "weight loss popularity scale"—and you are surely familiar with them: Low Carb (LC) and Intermittent Fasting (IF). Both deserve a brief special chapter for this very reason—so that you have good arguments for the next weight loss small talk, when someone inevitably says: "Yes, but intermittent fasting, and especially low carb, those definitely make you slim in the long run, I've read so much about it…"

U. Knop, *Successful and Sustainable Weight Loss*,
https://doi.org/10.1007/978-3-662-72477-4_2

2.1 Low Carb (LC) and Intermittent Fasting (IF)

LC is a very old and long-promoted "elimination diet" in which the body's main source of energy is more or less strictly omitted: carbohydrates such as bread, pasta, rice, sugar, and wheat flour, which now bear the stigma of being "harmful, unhealthy fatteners," must be removed from the plate. In IF, on the other hand, no specific foods are excluded; instead, much longer intervals are left between meals, so you only eat during these "intervals."

Let's be brief: For Low Carb (LC) and Intermittent Fasting (IF), there are neither official, standardized definitions nor scientific evidence that people lose weight more effectively with these dietary approaches than with any other diet. Nor are there any long-term studies or evidence (proof) for the form of ongoing, non-weight-loss-related nutrition practiced by many people, showing that LC or IF promotes health, protects against disease, or extends life—let alone that they can be "specifically used as the best nutritional therapy."

2.2 Myth of LC: Neither Makes You Slim(mer) Nor Healthy

Especially in the latter case, it is often claimed that improvements in certain "surrogate parameters"—that is, substitute values when there are no hard endpoints such as heart attacks or strokes, for example, blood values or similar—are a direct effect of LC or IF. But this is a misconception, because in the end, these improved parameters are generally always the result of (sometimes substantial) weight loss—and the body does not care which calorie-restricted diet forced it to lose fat. A good example was presented by scientists from the Essen-Mitte Clinics at the autumn congress of the DDG (German Diabetes Association) (Geissel 2017): With an extreme diet of less than 1000 kcal on so-called carbohydrate days, 70% of diabetics were able to improve their severe insulin resistance—and this was achieved with high carb (HC), i.e., primarily carbohydrates, not with the LC diet, to which this effect is often attributed by LC advocates.

Especially in the field of diet comparison studies—some of which you are already familiar with from the previous chapter—numerous publications have consistently delivered the same result: It makes no difference whether weight loss is achieved with LC or HC; the short-term "successes" are comparable. For example, the DIETFITS study, a randomized clinical trial conducted at the highest medical standards and published in the top journal *JAMA* (Gardner et al. 2018), confirmed this finding:

> The weight loss effect of an LC diet among the 609 overweight or obese participants was comparable to that of a low-fat diet after twelve months.

Regardless, there are of course plenty of advocates and promoters of LC who tirelessly proclaim the superiority of LC wherever possible. But—those who read carefully will also notice the following: Alongside the myth of LC as a weight loss miracle, there is a growing number of voices and studies that deny this dietary approach any health-promoting effects; here are a few selected original headlines from relevant articles in the German-language professional and popular press: "High-protein diet increases risk of heart failure" (2018a), "Carbohydrate restriction can be very risky in diabetes" (Klein 2018), "Study: Low-carbohydrate diet may shorten lifespan" (2018c), "Low-Carb—The Diet Lie" (Stern 2018).

And the renowned American professional society

American College of Cardiology issued a press release on the occasion of a recent study based on data from the National Institutes of Health, in which the study authors made it clear that "low-carb diets are associated with cardiac arrhythmias" (Napoli 2019). These findings also concerned the German Association of Internists, which likewise published its own press release (BDI 2019): "Low-carb diets increase the risk of atrial fibrillation. Those who consume too few carbohydrates are more likely to develop atrial fibrillation." The long-term effects of low-carbohydrate diets remain controversial, especially regarding their impact on cardiovascular disease, warned Dr. Xiaodong Zhuang, lead author of the study and cardiologist at Sun Yat-sen University Hospital. In view of the possible influence on arrhythmias, their study suggested that this popular method of weight control should be recommended with caution. One possible explanation is that increased consumption of protein and fat instead of carbohydrates triggers oxidative stress, which may also be related to atrial fibrillation.

The German Society of Cardiology (DGK) was particularly explicit, issuing the following press release on the occasion of the European Cardiology Congress (Fleck 2018): "Low-carb diets are dangerous and should be avoided. People on long-term low-carb diets have an increased risk of premature death, and their risks for causes of death such as heart disease, stroke, and cancer are also elevated." Certainly, the authors here, too, have somewhat over-interpreted the causal implications based on observational studies (more on this in Chap. 16)—however, the data underlying the DGK's statement certainly show no positive effects of LC on health or longevity.

Once again, the authors (free from conflicts of interest) of a major review (Brouns 2018), published in the *European Journal of Nutrition*, point out the usual knowledge gaps regarding the key question: "Overweight and diabetes prevention: Is a low-carbohydrate, high-fat diet advisable?" The answers are clear, since the data are unclear: "Due to the complexity of the potential mechanisms underlying LC, their interactions, and the lack of data from strictly controlled long-term studies (longer than 2 years), a general evidence-based recommendation of LCHF diets as a preventive measure to reduce the risk of type 2 diabetes seems premature. There is a lack of data demonstrating the long-term efficacy, safety, and health compatibility of LCHF (LowCarbHighFat) diets. Any LC recommendation should take this lack of evidence into account." And then comes the favorite closing sentence of all nutrition studies:

> "Low-carbohydrate diets require further investigation before general recommendations can be made."

A research group from the American cardiovascular society NLA (National Lipid Association) reached almost identical conclusions in the *Journal of Clinical Lipology*. This scientific statement provides a comprehensive overview of the current evidence base, drawn from recent systematic reviews and meta-analyses on the effects of low- and very-low-carbohydrate diets, including on body weight. The cardiology experts state clearly:

> "Based on the evidence reviewed, low- and very-low-carbohydrate diets are not superior to other dietary approaches for weight loss."

There are only minimal data on long-term efficacy and safety (>2 years). The American researchers also make a clear recommendation to their medical colleagues: "Physicians are encouraged to consider the findings discussed in this scientific statement when counseling patients about LC diets" (Kirckpatrick et al. 2019).

2.3 Criticism of LC Grows Louder

The Association for Independent Health Counseling (UGB) even dedicated an entire special issue of its journal UGB-forum to carbohydrate and LC myths, titled "Carbohydrates Controversial" (UGB 2018)—with a clear message: "Low-carb diets such as the Logi method, paleo, or ketogenic diets are promoted as health-enhancing by numerous self-help authors, in the media, and on social networks. Yet, current research still provides no evidence that reducing carbohydrates is sustainably beneficial to health."

The same applies, incidentally, to the "alternative energy source" for carbohydrates in LC diets—fat—since LC typically involves higher fat consumption. A group of authors in the journal *Science* (Ludwig et al. 2018) reached a clear conclusion on the question "How much fat is actually healthy?"—for the editorial team of the German Press Agency (dpa), this conclusion amounted to a …

> "… declaration of bankruptcy: Current evidence suggests that no specific carbohydrate-to-fat ratio in the diet is optimal for the general population."

Moreover, not all diets and calorie sources have similar metabolic effects in all individuals (dpa 2018). That's how it is.

This is also the view of Prof. Stefan Lorkowski, Head of Nutritional Biochemistry at the University of Jena: "It is certainly appealing, but naïve, to believe that simply changing the ratio of carbohydrates to fats is sufficient. What matters far more is their nutritional quality and, above all, the energy balance" (Ärzteblatt 2019). This central aspect is also confirmed by Prof. Alfred Wirth, former president of the German Obesity Society: "Almost all studies show that a low-carb diet is not superior and that, above all, the energy deficit is decisive for weight loss" (Wirth 2018). Both Lorkowski and Wirth consider the increase in LDL cholesterol with LC diets to be a health concern; Wirth also points to the stimulation of pro-inflammatory factors as a further critical aspect of LC diets.

These LC-contra statements could fill many more pages (just like the LC-pro studies—that's the "beauty" for all the nutrition gurus), but let's leave it at that—for now. However, let's give the final word to former DGE president Prof. Helmut Heseker with a prognosis: "The long-hyped low-carb diets are now losing their mass appeal and fascination. The years-long demonization of carbohydrates is suddenly being exposed by trendsetters as a major error. Atkins, South Beach, Hollywood Star, Mayo, Logi, and Paleo diets—regardless of evolution or Harvard—are not only being revealed as ineffective, but worse: previously overlooked or denied side effects (including bad breath, muscle cramps, nausea, and headaches) are now coming to the fore." (Heseker 2019)

2.4 Intermittent Fasting—Evidence-Free Eating-Free Time Windows

Even more dominant in terms of "media presence and celebrity promotion" is, and remains to this day (mid-2025), intermittent fasting (IF). And just as there is no clear official definition for LC, none of the various, entirely invented IF concepts can claim their own "personal creation" as the "best of IF." Thus, you find daily IF variations like 5:2 or 6:1, meaning you can eat whatever, whenever, and as much as you want on the first number of days, and "fast" (more or less strictly) on the second number of days. The 6:1 version even made it into the top five "celebrity diets to avoid in 2017," as selected annually by the British Dietetic Association.

The 6:1 diet is essentially a softer version of the 5:2 diet, both of which—no surprise—promise equal success in weight loss and health. The basic idea is always the same: by abstaining from food, the IF practitioner is supposed to save a significant portion of weekly calories on the "fasting days" and thus lose weight. But this is wishful thinking: In the end—or rather, at the end of the week, month, and especially the year—only one factor determines our weight: the overall energy balance. The body loses weight if, over the medium to long term, you consume fewer calories than you expend (negative energy balance). And that's where the real problem lies. If you eat more on the other days than you save on the fasting days, you certainly won't lose weight. You might even gain weight. And, on top of that, you may develop a mild eating disorder due to the constant decoupling of eating from natural hunger cues on the "fasting days."

For those who find one or two days of fasting too "hardcore," the diet gurus naturally have an appropriate IF solution: simply incorporate longer meal breaks into your daily routine. Here, the numbers refer to hours, not days. Typically, you skip one meal a day so that you go 16 or 14 hours without eating. In the remaining eight or ten hours, you are allowed to eat. Well, that's still plenty of time to eat. Not so with the extreme IF trend from the USA: the OMAD diet (One Meal A Day) is considered the hardcore version of intermittent fasting—here, the 23:1 hour principle dominates. You have to eat a lot in one hour to avoid starving in the long run.

Joking aside: As is typical, there is a lack of long-term data and evidence for IF showing that this form of "special eating" leads to better weight loss, improved health, or even to fewer "hard endpoints" (the gold standard scientific parameters) such as fewer heart attacks, strokes, or reduced mortality. And just as there are many studies with positive results (short-term data and surrogate markers), there are also critical papers and statements, which have also been reported in the media:

Foremost among these was a paper published in one of the most prestigious medical journals, which even ranked among the top ten most discussed medical articles published in 2020 in *JAMA Internal Medicine*. Fittingly, its sobering negative IF results were covered by nearly all media outlets—the headlines were essentially always the same: "Why Intermittent Fasting Doesn't Work/IF Alone Is Not the Solution/IF Doesn't Help with Weight Loss/IF Is No Panacea for Obesity/Intermittent Fasting Apparently Not an Effective Slimming Method?/IF Even Unhealthy?" That's just a small selection; the headlines could fill pages. What "happened"? The US researchers investigated the 16:8 IF concept in their randomized controlled trial (Lowe et al. 2020). The overweight participants lost about 1 kg (approximately 1% of their initial body weight) within 12 weeks, but: No significant difference was documented compared to the control group, who ate their three main meals in the usual morning-noon-evening rhythm. There were also no significant differences between the groups in insulin and blood sugar levels or other laboratory values. However, one striking difference emerged: the intermittent fasting group lost significantly more muscle mass than the comparison group—this loss was even greater than the muscle loss typically seen with diets. But that is exactly what you want to avoid when losing weight—the goal is primarily to lose "dangerous internal (visceral) abdominal fat." Unfortunately, this number one weight loss target seems resistant to IF … because just as the media coverage of the aforementioned *JAMA* study subsided, another paper with concerning results appeared: IF apparently does not help against harmful visceral fat, as it remains stubborn and resists breakdown. Researchers found that a key protein in abdominal fat responsible for fat breakdown was reduced fourfold. And that wasn't all: "Unfortunately," the proportion of molecules responsible for building visceral fat cells actually increased (Harney et al. 2021).

However, these studies were by no means the first of their kind; many years earlier, numerous negative papers on IF had already been reported: "Obesity: Intermittent fasting in a randomized clinical trial (published in JAMA) shows no benefits—the dropout rate was even higher than with conventional calorie restriction" (Ärzteblatt 2017), "Intermittent fasting is not a fountain of youth" (Scinexx 2017), "The findings on intermittent fasting are almost all based on animal studies—there are no limits to arbitrariness or commercial interests" (Bartens 2018), and "The current trend toward intermittent fasting lacks a scientific basis" (Zinkant 2018), "Does intermittent fasting promote the development of type 2 diabetes?" (Ärzteblatt 2018b), and "Intermittent fasting may facilitate weight loss, but does not improve metabolism" (Ärzteblatt 2018d), "There are only a few studies on intermittent fasting so far. In particular, studies with sufficiently large sample sizes and long-term data are lacking" (Verbraucherzentrale Bayern 2018).

Researchers at the German Cancer Research Center and Heidelberg University Hospital addressed this data gap and conducted their HELENA study, the largest investigation to date (RCT, randomized controlled trial) on IF (Schübel 2018)—with the following results, which were widely communicated in a press release (Koh 2018):

"Intermittent fasting: No advantage over conventional diets. In both diet groups, participants lost visceral fat along with body weight—that is, the unhealthy abdominal fat—as well as fat deposits in the liver." The researchers also found no differences between the two diet forms in any of the other metabolic parameters analyzed, nor in any of the biomarkers or gene activities studied. While the HELENA study does not support the euphoric expectations for intermittent fasting, it also showed that this method is not inferior to a conventional diet. Prof. Tilman Kühn, lead scientist of the study, interprets the results as follows:

> "The key is not the type of diet, but rather choosing a method and sticking with it."

He further explains: "This is also suggested by a recent study comparing low-carb and low-fat diets—that is, reducing carbohydrates versus reducing fat while otherwise maintaining a balanced diet. Here, too, participants achieved comparable effects with both methods." This comparison refers to the previously mentioned DIETFITS study on low carb.

Ultimately, a pragmatic and liberal approach to nutrition is warranted here as well, in line with the essential message: "There are as many healthy diets as there are people, because everyone is different." So, if you do well with LC, go ahead and avoid carbohydrates. If you have found your "culinary gold standard" in 5:2, 6:1, or X:X IF, that's great. But if you neither can nor want to give up carbohydrates, nor are a fan of fasting for hours or days, you need not worry that you are eating "less healthily" or losing weight less effectively. That is nothing more than pure populism.

LC and IF are probably so popular because both of these "better-eating hypes" are very easy to implement, as there are no complicated rules or elaborate calculations. "It works quite well because, for many people, it is probably easier to completely give up something than to always pay close attention to their diet. In my experience, people find black-and-white easier than gray," explained Dr. Gert Bischoff, a nutrition physician from Munich, on Bayerischer Rundfunk BR, regarding the "success" of IF (Keller 2018).

No plea *against* LC and IF!

To make it absolutely clear: This chapter is *not* a plea against LC and IF. Its purpose is simply to show you that even publicly hyped diet forms are not better than other weight loss approaches. It is meant to relieve the pressure to "absolutely try LC or IF because they are so popular and incredibly successful." However, for people who naturally do not care much for carbohydrates, LC can be a very viable way to choose foods. And IF has the great advantage that it allows true, biological hunger to be fully experienced—a very important physiological process that not only initiates numerous positive metabolic effects but also ensures full enjoyment of eating. After all, without hunger, a meal does not taste as good as it could and should (see also Chap. 18). For Harald Seitz, spokesperson for the Federal Center for Nutrition (BZfE) and nutrition scientist, IF is even "the simplest method to lose weight," because "it is relatively easy to implement. You know when you are allowed to eat and when not. And in principle, you can eat whatever you want. You don't need new recipes." With diets, you have to watch out for deficiencies, but with IF the risk is low "because you are basically allowed to eat everything" (Hasse 2021). And this is something IF shares with the individual approach I DIET MY WAY, which you will learn more about later in this book: You may and should eat whatever you want. But more on that later. And then it's up to you: Decide freely, al gusto! Because "when it comes to losing weight, the main thing is to consume less energy and expend more. Not to follow a specific diet," explains Prof. Dr. Hartmut Bertz, senior physician and head of the Section of Nutritional Medicine and Dietetics at the University Medical Center Freiburg, describing the "hypocaloric universal principle" of any weight reduction (Faßnacht-Lee 2021).

Key Points of the Chapter

LC and IF have much in common: There are neither official definitions nor long-term evidence for hard endpoints, nor scientific proof that these particular ways of eating are healthier than any other dietary pattern. Furthermore, there are no valid data demonstrating superiority in terms of improved weight loss. In short: LC and IF do not make you slimmer than conventional diets with comparable calorie reduction. If you like them, great; if not, don't worry! The motto for achieving and maintaining your desired weight is: I DIET MY WAY … and how you find your way is what comes next. Wishing you a good journey to your new, slimmer self …

2.5 Summary: Your Current State of Knowledge

At this point in your journey to your new desired weight, you now know …

- All diets are based on the same principle: negative energy balance.
- There is no better or worse diet—all diets are equal.
- Most weight loss programs fail and lead to weight gain, as they are both impersonal and not tailored to the individual, and are only followed for a short time.
- The result: the vicious circle/circulus vitiosus:
  (new) diet fails ➔ weight gain ➔ fear of failure/self-doubt ➔ (new) diet fails ➔ …
- Classical diets are therefore considered a "gateway drug" to eating disorders and obesity.
- **Even trendy diets like low carb and intermittent fasting are not better than other diets, no matter what the media, influencers, and celebrities write and post.**

References

Ärzteblatt (2017) Adipositas: Intervallfasten in klinischer Studie ohne Vorteile. https://www.aerzteblatt.de/nachrichten/74460/Adipositas-Intervallfasten-in-klinischer-Studie-ohne-Vorteile. Accessed: 5. Sept. 2020

Ärzteblatt (2018a, Mai 30) Ernährung: Eiweißdiät erhöht Risiko auf Herzinsuffizienz. https://www.aerzteblatt.de/nachrichten/95518/Ernaehrung-Eiweissdiaet-erhoeht-Risiko-auf-Herzinsuffizienz. Accessed: 5. Sept. 2020

Ärzteblatt (2018b, Juni 12) Begünstigt Intervallfasten die Entwicklung eines Typ-2-Diabetes? https://www.aerzteblatt.de/blog/95375/Beguenstigt-Intervallfasten-die-Entwicklung-eines-Typ-2-Diabetes. Accessed: 5. Sept. 2020

Ärzteblatt (2018c, August 17) Studie: Kohlenhydratarme Ernährung kann Leben verkürzen. https://www.aerzteblatt.de/nachrichten/97232/Studie-Kohlenhydratarme-Ernaehrung-kann-Leben-verkuerzen-ausser-bei-Vegetariern. Accessed: 5. Sept. 2020

Ärzteblatt (2018d, November 26) Intervallfasten kann Gewichtsabnahme erleichtern, verbessert aber nicht den Stoffwechsel. https://www.aerzteblatt.de/nachrichten/99412/Intervallfasten-kann-Gewichtsabnahme-erleichtern-verbessert-aber-nicht-den-Stoffwechsel. Accessed: 5. Sept. 2020

Ärzteblatt (2019) Pro und Contra: Sind Low-Carb-Diäten zur Therapie von Übergewicht und Diabetes geeignet? https://www.aerzteblatt.de/nachrichten/100250/Pro-und-Contra-Sind-Low-Carb-Diaeten-zur-Therapie-von-Uebergewicht-und-Diabetes-geeignet#comments. Accessed: 5. Sept. 2020

Bartens W (2018) Ein neuer Diättrend. https://www.tagesanzeiger.ch/leben/essen-und-trinken/gewichtiger-einwand/story/23524614. Accessed: 5. Sept. 2020

BDI (2019) Bei Low-Carb-Ernährung droht mehr Vorhofflimmern. https://www.internisten-im-netz.de/aktuelle-meldungen/aktuell/bei-low-carb-ernaehrung-droht-mehr-vorhofflimmern.html. Accessed: 5. Sept. 2020

Brouns F (2018) Overweight and diabetes prevention: is a low-carbohydrate–high-fat diet recommendable? Eur J Nutr 57:1301–1312. https://doi.org/10.1007/s00394-018-1636-y

dpa (2018) Wie viel Fett gehört zu einer gesunden Ernährung? https://www.ksta.de/ratgeber/wie-viel-fett-gehoert-zu-einer-gesunden-ernaehrung%2D%2D32182008. Accessed: 5. Sept. 2020

Faßnacht-Lee K (2021) Ketogene Diät: Gesund oder gefährlich? https://www.aponet.de/artikel/ketogene-diaet-gesund-oder-gefaehrlich-23113. Accessed on 15.02.2021

Fleck E (2018) Low-Carb-Ernährung ist gefährlich und sollte gemieden werden. https://idw-online.de/en/news701236. Accessed: 5. Sept. 2020

Gardner D et al (2018) Effect of low-fat vs low-carbohydrate diet on 12-month weight loss in overweight adults and the association with genotype pattern or insulin secretion. The DIETFITS randomized clinical trial. JAMA 319(7):667–679. https://doi.org/10.1001/jama.2018.0245

Geissel W (2017) Typ-2-Diabetes. Mit Kohlenhydrat-Tagen die Insulinresistenz durchbrechen. https://www.aerztezeitung.de/Medizin/Mit-Kohlenhydrat-Tagen-die-Insulinresistenz-durchbrechen-309497.html. Accessed: 5. Sept. 2020

Harney et al (2021) Proteomics analysis of adipose depots after intermittent fasting reveals visceral fat preservation mechanisms. Cell Rep 34. https://doi.org/10.1016/j.celrep.2021.108804. Accessed on 14.03.2021

Hasse T (2021) Ernährung und Abnehmen – Intervallfasten: Jede Stunde zählt. https://www.deutschlandfunknova.de/beitrag/intervallfasten-abnehmen-ohne-kalorien-zaehlen. Accessed on 17.01.2021

Heseker H (2019) Nachschlag: Über Aufstieg und Fall von Ernährungshypes. https://www.ernaehrungs-umschau.de/news/09-5-2019-ueber-aufstieg-und-fall-von-ernaehrungshypes/. Accessed: 5. Sept. 2020

Keller V (2018) Intervallfasten – Abnehmen mit dem Ernährungstrend? https://www.br.de/br-fernsehen/sendungen/gesundheit/intervallfasten-ernaehrung-abnehmen-100.html. Accessed: 5. Sept. 2020

Kirckpatrick et al (2019) Review of current evidence and clinical recommendations on the effects of low-carbohydrate and very-low-carbohydrate (including ketogenic) diets for the management of body weight and other cardiometabolic risk factors: a scientific statement from the National Lipid Association Nutrition and Lifestyle Task Force. J Clin Lipidol. https://doi.org/10.1016/j.jacl.2019.08.003

Klein F (2018) Kohlenhydratverzicht kann bei Diabetes sehr riskant sein. https://www.medical-tribune.de/medizin-und-forschung/artikel/kohlenhydratverzicht-kann-bei-diabetes-sehr-riskant-sein/. Accessed: 5. Sept. 2020

Koh (2018) Intervallfasten: Kein Vorteil gegenüber herkömmlichen Diäten. https://www.dkfz.de/de/presse/pressemitteilungen/2018/dkfz-pm-18-64-Intervallfasten-Kein-Vorteil-gegenueber-herkoemmlichen-Diaeten.php. Accessed: 5. Sept. 2020

Lowe et al (2020) Effects of time-restricted eating on weight loss and other metabolic parameters in women and men with overweight and obesity. The TREAT randomized clinical trial. JAMA Intern Med. 180(11):1491–1499. https://doi.org/10.1001/jamainternmed.2020.4153

Ludwig et al (2018) Dietary fat: from foe to friend? Science 362(6416):764–770. https://doi.org/10.1126/science.aau2096

Napoli N (2019) Low-carb diet tied to common heart rhythm disorder. https://www.acc.org/about-acc/press-releases/2019/03/06/10/29/low-carb-diet-tied-to-common-heart-rhythm-disorder. Accessed: 5. Sept. 2020

Schübel R (2018) Effects of intermittent and continuous calorie restriction on body weight and metabolism over one year: a randomized controlled trial. Am J Clin Nutr. https://doi.org/10.1093/ajcn/nqy196

Scinexx (2017) Intervallfasten taugt nicht als Jungbrunnen. https://www.scinexx.de/news/biowissen/intervallfasten-taugt-nicht-als-jungbrunnen/. Accessed: 5. Sept. 2020

Stern (2018) Low-Carb – Die Diäten-Lüge. https://www.stern.de/gesundheit/low-carb-die-diaeten-luege-3540996.html. Accessed: 5. Sept. 2020

UGB (2018) Kohlenhydrate kontrovers. UGBforum 4/2018. https://www.ugb.de/images/ugb-forum/2018/4-kohlenhydrate/inhalt-4-18.pdf. Accessed: 5. Sept. 2020

Verbraucherzentrale Bayern (2018) Intervallfasten. https://projekte.meine-verbraucherzentrale.de/DE-BY/intervallfasten. Accessed: 5. Sept. 2020

Wirth A (2018) Low Carb zum Abnehmen: Lust oder Frust? CV 18:56. https://doi.org/10.1007/s15027-018-1484-y

Zinkant K (2018) Von Mäusen und Hüftgold. https://www.sueddeutsche.de/wissen/diaet-intervallfasten-ratgeber-wissenschaft-1.4268786?reduced=true. Accessed: 5. Sept. 2020

3 Reset Your Mindset: Who Am I and What Do I Want?

Before you embark on your own personal "Get Slim Project," you should clarify some essential questions with yourself—and be completely honest and sincere in the process. When you take on such a significant life challenge of enormous consequence, the foundation on which it stands must be rock solid. Weak points based on uncertainty or even "self-deception" can cause your entire life goal to collapse like a house of cards. In this spirit: the truth, and nothing but the truth. Let's begin …

… with a kind of "characterization of weight-loss types," to find out: Where do you see yourself, to which "class" do you belong?

Overview: Weight-Loss Types

Naturally Slim

Can eat and drink whatever they want and do not gain weight. Do not need to exercise to stay slim.

Goal: Want to become even thinner.

Important to note: Avoid becoming too "emaciated" and ensure sufficient nutrient intake if eating very little.

U. Knop, *Successful and Sustainable Weight Loss*,
https://doi.org/10.1007/978-3-662-72477-4_3

Normal Weight
Need to pay some attention to their diet, and typically gain weight gradually over the course of life. Look relatively normal, but not truly slim. Are bothered here and there by a few extra kilos of fat on their body.

Goal: Want to lose a few kilos, preferably in specific "problem areas."

Important to note: Nothing special beyond the correct long-term adjustment of diet and lifestyle (that is, what you will read and learn throughout this book).

Overweight (Mild to Moderate)
Often need to pay (very) close attention to their diet to avoid further weight gain. Usually not a health concern, but socially classified as "too heavy." Consequently, they feel too fat. Especially in a bikini or swim trunks.

Goal: Want to lose weight visibly and significantly.

Important to note: Nothing special beyond the correct long-term adjustment of diet and lifestyle.

Genetically Obese (Naturally Obese)
Are very heavy, obese due to genetics. Just looking at food seems to make them "gain a kilo instantly." Even when they eat little, they lose weight only very slowly because they are efficient "food processors" and well insulated (= energy efficient).

Goal: Want to be of normal weight or only slightly overweight, so they are no longer looked at reproachfully when out in public (especially when eating).

Important to note: Significant and lasting weight reduction in this group is often only achievable—if at all—with "bariatric assistance" (surgical weight-loss procedures, such as gastric banding), because: you can't "turn a St. Bernard into a greyhound." With tremendous willpower and an unwavering desire for change, a few manage it "without the scalpel." However, after rapid weight loss, excess skin often remains, which may need to be surgically removed.

"Emotionally Overweight"
Are actually biologically slimmer, but have "eaten up" their natural body weight due to frustration, and are unnaturally heavy because of emotional eating (eating without hunger out of frustration, sorrow, boredom, grief, dissatisfaction, stress, anxiety, loneliness—to feed the soul and calm the psyche).

Goal: Regain control over eating, "defeat" emotional eating, and lose weight to return to their former figure.

Important to note: Identify the true reasons for emotional overeating, address them at the root, and eliminate the causes from your life.

Because: here, eating is not the reason for being overweight, but rather the physical/emotional causes that lead to feeding the soul without physical hunger.

Diet-Induced Overweight
After several diets that were briefly successful, have always regained the weight, so that both starting weight and body fat percentage are significantly higher than before beginning their "diet career"—the classic yo-yo body, heavier and with more fat (emergency reserves) than before, possibly also with a reduced basal metabolic rate (the body has activated an energy-saving mode).

Goal: Escape the yo-yo trap and finally maintain the reduced weight permanently.

Important to note: The next dietary and lifestyle adaptation should be the last—it must fit completely with both the person and their personality, as well as with family and work life, so that it can be maintained long-term and for life.

Pathologically/Metabolically Obese
Suffer from a physical/organic illness that, due to metabolic disturbance (e.g., thyroid/cortisone) and/or medications, has caused them to become overweight—or are obese due to psychological disorders/eating disorders. The cause could also be a mental illness such as depression or a physical fat distribution disorder.

Goal: Become healthy (if possible) in order to lose weight.

Important to note: Before undertaking a planned, significantly calorie-reduced dietary change, be sure to consult a doctor and discuss the plan together, so that the therapy or therapies are not undermined.

Miscellaneous Overweight
An individual blend of numerous "minor" reasons that together have gradually led to becoming overweight, for example: stress, eating disorders, medications, lack of physical activity, sleep deprivation/poor sleep quality, social problems, quitting smoking ...

Goal: Dissolve the "overweight mix," break the vicious cycle, and return to a naturally biological normal figure.

Important to note: The detailed "adipogenic history" is the focus—in other words: Which causes contribute to increasing body weight, and how? How can these first be untangled and then resolved?

Special Category: Power Woman
A particularly tall and strongly built woman, such as Brienne of Tarth from the hit series "Game of Thrones." Stands out visually due to her "superwoman" proportions.

Goal: Wants to look and appear overall more feminine and graceful, and less masculine.

Important to note: The slim silhouette is often naturally and biologically limited by bone structure and skeletal build.

3.1 Short Thinking and Reflection Break

Before we continue, here comes probably the most important question: Why are the kilos where they are, when I actually don't want them there? The following brief meditative reflection guide will help you find some initial answers on the spot, to see which of the aforementioned categories you identify with.

Mini-Meditation for Initial Self-Insight

Make yourself comfortable and create a pleasant space where you feel at ease. Sit down, feet on the floor, back as straight as possible. Breathe deeply into your abdomen, about a hand's width below your navel. Allow your core, your belly, to expand freely as you inhale; don't hold anything back and relax. Exhale slowly and evenly. Close your eyes and repeat this breathing two or three times. Now ask yourself (out loud): "Why do I have these extra kilos? Are they there to protect me emotionally?" Listen carefully to what they are protecting you from. Did they arise out of boredom? Does my body actually want to be nourished differently and has therefore accumulated them? Am I emotionally out of balance somewhere, so that I need the kilos as a counterweight? Be completely honest with yourself here, because: Everything is okay, everything is allowed, and it helps you to understand yourself better in the future and to be able to adjust more quickly. If you experience one of your own answers as a real feeling for the first time, so intensely that it touches you deeply and makes you sad or brings you to tears—then let it happen and become aware that your body (probably) wanted to protect you with its extra kilos. And with this question that makes you sad/emotional, you are exactly on the right track. You can and should now integrate this realization into your upcoming solution strategies. To conclude, thank your body and tell it: "In the future, we won't need the extra kilos anymore, because I will make sure that we are well—or even better: better off!"

So, are you a little wiser now? What do you think: Which of the weight loss types do you belong to? It's important to become clear about this, because each of the different "kilo-killer classes" requires specific, appropriately focused lifestyle adaptations. In the following, we will not explicitly present a very specific hypocaloric (energy-deficient) diet for each of the types listed above. Firstly, because there are, of course, numerous mixed forms, overlaps, and entirely individual blends of the above types—and certainly some "exotic classes" not mentioned here—and secondly, because the fundamental principle of sustainable weight loss always remains the same at its core. So if you're now asking yourself: "Yes, then what is the point of all this typology?"—then you're asking the right question.

The answer is simple. Because in addition to the universal principle of weight loss, it is also clear: All the different weight loss types have "specialties" that absolutely must be taken into account. The essential aspects are therefore listed directly above. You can then pursue this "thought starter" further for yourself: For example, if you primarily identify with the "emotional eaters," then your focus should be on "psychological hygiene," working through the emotional issues that lead to emotional eating. Why is the psyche being appeased with calories? What triggers lead to compensatory eating? Many more questions arise just within this topic alone—for which entire single-topic books could be written (and surely exist). If you now know this about yourself and your character, perhaps even for the first time in your life due to your honest self-reflection, then you can now address it—and you should, in order to achieve long-term success in losing weight. This can be a supporting or a dominant factor, depending on how important and relevant this realization is for your life.

Or, as another example, if you are morbidly obese, then it is of course extremely important to first get healthy or, at the very least, to discuss your desire to lose weight not only with your treating physician but also to "synchronize" this path very closely with your therapy—you should not do this on your own! Here, medicine and nutrition must be closely interlinked as part of a multimodal therapy. But that is another "chapter" that will not be further addressed here. Because:

3.2 "I Am Healthy and Want to Lose Weight!"

This book is written only for people who are fundamentally healthy and want to lose weight and reach a new desired weight on their own, without professional external/medical help. I want to accompany and guide you on this journey. So, after you have reflected and recognized which weight loss type you are, we can now move on to the next "core questions before the weight loss project." The focus here is on the following:

> **Note**
>
> **RESET your MINDSET!**
>
> **Who am I? What does it feel like to live in this body and to be the way I am?**

At the beginning stands the "click moment for lifestyle modification" in your mind, or in modern terms, mindset—formerly called mentality, meaning your personal way of thinking and inner attitude. Successful weight loss begins in the mind. Specifically: You need to be clear and become aware:

- Who am I, what does it feel like to live in this body and to be who I am?
- And then the question arises: Where do I want to go—and what do I want and what do I **no longer** want?
- Where am I in life, what role does my weight play in my life?
- What do I do and, above all, what do I **not** do because of my weight—and what am I unable to do because of my body size, but would love to?
- What do I need to "reprogram in my mindset," in my head, what is going wrong, what do I need and **want** to change?
- What goals and wishes do I see in weight reduction? And above all:

> Uncover your inner motivation: Why, honestly, do you want to lose weight? And how many kilos do you want to lose permanently, and where?

3.3 And the Switch Has Flipped—Turn It On!

Be aware: If you want to lose weight, that means: I will most likely have to suffer as well! And: You need time, you must be patient and understanding with yourself—because there will also be setbacks or times of "reduction stagnation," meaning that suddenly nothing happens with weight loss. Losing weight sustainably and permanently, and above all staying slim and maintaining your new weight, takes time—sometimes several years, depending on your starting point. But only then is there the highest probability of keeping your new slim self and making it your new body. Losing weight is a lifelong task, a challenge that both men and women must face fully "with body and soul."

Your goal should not be to lose weight to please other people or to meet current beauty ideals—which, in any case, are usually only permanently achievable with Photoshop. Because that can quickly lead to failure. You have to want it and do it for yourself: The "game changer" is you! Your own goal should be to find and maintain your personal desired and feel-good weight in the long term—as well as to stay fit, healthy, and in the best of spirits. Here, it's important to find a healthy balance between restrictions and moments of enjoyment. In this spirit …

This is exactly the challenge we are now taking on. Or rather: you are.

The Most Important Points of the Chapter

- Be fully aware
  - who you are, why you want what you want, and what your goals are,
  - why your body looks the way it does and where the kilos come from.
- Your first "mini psychoanalysis" must be **honest and sincere**.
- Set your mindset to "start into your new slim self"—flip the switch!

3.4 Summary: Your Current State of Knowledge

At this point in your journey toward your desired weight, you now know …

- All diets are based on the same principle: a negative energy balance.
- There is no better or worse diet—all diets are the same.
- Most weight loss programs fail and actually lead to weight gain, as they are both impersonal, not tailored to the individual, and only carried out for a short period of time.
- The result: the vicious circle/circulus vitiosus:
  (new) diet fails ➔ weight gain ➔ fear of failure/self-doubt ➔ (new) diet fails ➔ …
- Classic diets are therefore considered a "gateway drug" to eating disorders and obesity.
- Trendy diets like low carb and intermittent fasting are also no better than other diets, no matter what the media, influencers, and celebrities write and post.
- **My new path begins with honest self-awareness: I need to be clear about who I am and what I want. My mindset must align with this. Then I can get started.**

4

Becoming Slim ... It's Not That Hard, Is It?!

Et voilà. Now you can get started. You know that off-the-shelf diets do not deliver what they promise—especially not "maintaining the new, slimmer weight." You also know your mindset and you know exactly what you want to achieve—and why. Now it's time to get down to the "nitty-gritty." You will now learn everything about the, at its core quite simple, physiological practice of losing weight as well as the essential basics that must always be considered when it comes to weight loss.

> "Whether and how much someone loses weight is always determined by the energy balance," says Hans Hauner, Professor of Nutritional Medicine at the Technical University of MuniChap. "Concepts that save 500 to 600 calories per day successfully reduce body weight." (test 2021)

U. Knop, *Successful and Sustainable Weight Loss*,
https://doi.org/10.1007/978-3-662-72477-4_4

4.1 Negative Energy Balance = Positive Weight Development

The above quote already summarizes the key findings well. Since you will probably never forget the negative energy balance, we will start this chapter directly with it—because it is the core of every diet: The fundamental element in losing weight is reducing your energy intake below the threshold of the calories your body needs per day, per week, per month—but: reduction without giving up something you enjoy eating. That is essential! Because only what you truly like should be part of the "essence of your diet," which you should not only eat every day, but also enjoy and celebrate this enjoyment. So, if you like eating carbohydrates, then low carb is the wrong approach for you—and keto even more so. If you enjoy meat, cheese, and the like, then don't do a vegetarian or even vegan diet—you will fail. You don't need to be "afraid" of unhealthy foods, because: They don't exist (more on this in Chaps. 16 and 17). For now, only one thing matters: Consume fewer calories than you burn. In principle, it's a very simple calculation. The current recommendations for sustainable "healthy" weight reduction are:

> The negative energy balance/calorie deficit should be minus 500 kcal per day.

This immediately raises two fundamental questions.

1. How much energy do I actually use on average per day?
2. How do I know how much I consume daily, and how do I save 500 kcal each day?

The first question is difficult to answer, because individual energy expenditure cannot be accurately analyzed or precisely measured, only estimated. This value depends on numerous factors that interact in very complex ways. Therefore, you should first start with the general average:

The average energy expenditure of a healthy woman is about 2000 kcal per day, that of a man about 2500 kcal.

Of course, it's clear: Those who do physical work all day and/or have to walk a lot will have significantly higher values. Conversely, those who mostly sit often have a lower value. Therefore, it is important that you personally decide which baseline value to start from. Average, a bit more, or less? Then you subtract 500 kcal from that every day. Sounds simple? It is. You just need to do a bit of research, documentation, and calculation. On the one hand, the calorie information is on the packaging—so if you cook and prepare food yourself, all you need is a pen and paper and the ability to do basic arithmetic and mental math. Or you can use a calculator. If you like to eat out, you have to rely on tables on the internet that give the approximate calorie content of a meal, trusting that a doner kebab with fries, a cheeseburger, a salami pizza, or whatever, has the corresponding calories. Many large fast food chains, for example, provide the values for all their products in detail. That is very helpful.

You do not necessarily have to save the 500 kcal every day. You can also cut them out cumulatively over two or three days at once—although this is tough on those extreme days, it provides more freedom and flexibility overall.

4.2 Obesity Guideline & The Calorie as a Guiding Unit

The significance and importance of focusing clearly on energy intake and calorie balance, rather than on specific diet plans, is also reflected in the new obesity guideline (AWMF 2024). This so-called S3 guideline is an "instruction manual" for physicians and therapists on how obese individuals should be treated so that they can lose weight sustainably and maintain the reduced weight. One of the main focuses is nutrition.

Recommended Diet in the S3 Guideline "Obesity"

To put it briefly: The new guideline does not recommend any specific diet—because there is no single optimal diet. The choice of dietary style should be made **individually** by the person wishing to lose weight, based on their eating habits, desires, and preferences. Obese individuals should therefore receive personalized, tailored dietary recommendations suited to their personal situation. Today, there are many scientifically well-studied ways to save dietary energy—so everyone should be able to find a dietary approach that suits them and makes it easier to manage their weight. Regardless of the dietary form, the fundamental goal is always a moderate **reduction in energy intake** while ensuring an adequate supply of essential (micro)nutrients. The aim is always a **long-term** change in diet—and this is only possible if the "new way of eating" appeals to the individual, tastes good, suits them, and makes them feel comfortable.

Only the Individual Path Leads to Success

According to the new S3 guideline, there is therefore no "one best diet." This is understandable, because, firstly: None of the many different diet trends such as **low carb, intermittent fasting, keto, paleo, vegan, clean eating & co.** is the best or healthiest. Furthermore, the scientific community now agrees, especially regarding the two "top diet trends" of recent years: Neither **low carb**—that is, largely avoiding carbohydrates—nor the popular **intermittent fasting** offer **any** advantages for weight loss compared to other calorie-reduced diets (as you know in detail from Chap. 2). Therefore, the dietary recommendations in the new obesity guideline are open and individualized—and not focused on one or two specific eating patterns.

Specific Recommendations of the New Guideline for "Obesity Therapy"

According to the updated guideline, the foundation of any obesity treatment—that is, the intended weight reduction—remains the "multimodal basic therapy," meaning an approach that considers several levels—specifically, the following three: dietary change, increased physical activity, and behavioral modification.

In terms of individualized nutrition and to achieve the fundamental goal of moderate **reduction in energy intake**, the following applies: Daily energy intake should be about 500 kilocalories (kcal) below daily requirements. This makes a weight loss of 0.5 kg per week over a period of three months realistic. At this point, we once again pose the specific question:

Why exactly 500 kcal less?

Prof. Hans Hauner from Munich, one of the coordinators of the new guideline, explains this number as follows: "This is a rough empirical (experiential knowledge) recommendation with which a moderate weight loss of 5 to 10% can be achieved. It is quite possible to save this amount of calories without giving overly strict recommendations or restricting the amount of food (which is essential for adequate satiety)" (Knop 2024). Moreover, no one needs to calculate their calorie requirements, because, as Hauner says: "We deliberately refrained from determining calorie requirements, because the usual formulas are quite inaccurate and even measurement by indirect calorimetry is subject to a relatively large margin of error. Instead, we recommend starting from the current diet and modifying it so that an energy deficit of this magnitude is achieved, without changing eating habits too drastically, which is difficult to sustain in the long term." But Hauner also cautions: "At best, there are only limited studies on this question, and there is actually a simple calculation logic behind it." And it looks like this:

1 kg of body fat corresponds to about 7000 kcal. Thus, the calculation is: 500 kcal less per day × 7 days = 3500 kcal/week "saved" = 0.5 kg less body fat = 500 g lost per week. This results in a moderate weight reduction of about 2 kg per month.

Is Calorie Counting Still Up to Date?

This is a topic of controversial debate today—not only physiologically, but also from a socio-historical perspective. Historian Dr. Nina Mackert from the University of Leipzig has conducted extensive research on this and views the 500-kcal saving recommendation in the new obesity guideline critically: "I consider this an illustrative example of how the logic of calorie counting upholds an image of individual nutrition in which individuals have their weight 'in their own hands' and can—and must—control it through supposedly 'correct' decisions. This very narrow view of healthy eating overlooks numerous influences that lie outside individual control."

It is the **product of a conception of the body that is by now long outdated from a historical perspective.** In addition, a larger body is depicted as a problem per se, and weight loss is equated with health, although this is partly disputed even in medical research (Knop 2024).

No question: One can and should view kilocalories critically today, as the scientific evidence is, in fact, not the strongest. But—and this is precisely why you will also find this 500-kcal benchmark in this book—this reference value can function as an **orientation value** in a weight loss concept. It is easy to work with, understandable, and fundamentally plausible. Therefore, the 500-kcal benchmark provides an initial corridor for the theoretical weight loss plan, aiming for healthy weight loss of about 500 g per week, to be implemented as part of an **individually adapted dietary and lifestyle change**—one that can be maintained in the long term. However, alternative approaches can also be chosen that do not require calorie counting. For example, both **Veganuary and Dry January** are not only trends at the start of the year, but also effective ways to lose weight—entirely without counting calories.

4.3 Veganuary and Dry January—Universally Harness the Potential of Omission!

By giving up meat, sausage, and alcohol, you can save up to 1000 kcal per day—without a calculator or app. Both abstaining from meat and sausage during **Veganuary** and giving up alcohol can significantly contribute to weight loss, as both food groups include a wide range of products, some with high calorie content. If you have regularly consumed both in substantial amounts until now, you will likely notice the effects of abstaining quite quickly on the scale. And all of this is child's play and immediately implementable—no meal plans, calorie counting, or other "challenges" required—just leave out certain foods and drinks and otherwise continue to eat just as deliciously as usual, done. And if you also eliminate or minimize sweets/snacks and soft drinks from your diet, the total calories saved can really add up.

Concrete numbers speak for themselves

The bare numbers alone are already impressive: If you just leave out sausage and meat, for example, on day 1, skipping a meal with a "missing" grilled bratwurst, that's about 800 kcal, and for a snack with 100 g cooked ham, another 100 kcal, totaling 900 kcal less. On the following day 2, it's the uneaten chicken breast or pork schnitzel, each saving about 400 kcal, plus the omitted salami at about 300 kcal (100g)—that's still a solid 700 kcal less.

If you now also skip the sweets/snacks, say on day 1 half a bar of chocolate and on day 2 50 g of chips, each at 250 kcal, that's a total of 1000 kcal less per day. Add to that a can of soft drink/cola at 150 kcal and ration out the alcohol (0.5 l beer 250 kcal or half a bottle of red wine 14% about 300 kcal or a can of "Jack Daniel's & Cola" about 300 kcal), and that's another 400 kcal not consumed. All the saved kilocalories add up to about 1500 kcal less per day!

This allows for real weight loss success, because ...

... the above calculation corresponds to half the daily requirement of a person doing moderate physical work (an "office worker" uses less). Such a worker would lose weight rapidly with such a massive negative energy balance. Even if these 1500 kcal are "replaced" with lots of vegetables, low-calorie carbohydrates, and cheese, and zero-calorie drinks are consumed—which together provide significantly less energy than meat, sausage, snacks, sweets, soft drinks, and alcohol—there still remains an energy deficit of about 500 kcal below requirements. And that is exactly the deficit recommended not only in the S3 guidelines of medical societies (see above), but also by many other independent institutions, such as Stiftung Warentest (test 2024), as a "moderate energy deficit for long-term healthy weight reduction," to lose about 500 g per week, i.e., about 2 kg per month. So it can be worthwhile to **continue with the new way of eating even after Veganuary**.

Start of the year: Let's get going!
If you truly want to bring your heartfelt wish "to become and stay slimmer" to life out of deep inner conviction, you can only lose about 2 kg per month in a healthy way through **individual dietary and lifestyle changes**. So if you want to have your best shape instead of a muffin top by summer, the good resolution is: Start right away in **Veganuary**! Before you begin, you should do a "personal tabula rasa": Turn your life thoroughly and completely upside down to intensely examine yourself and your own self: Who am I, why do I look the way I do, what do I want and what do I no longer want to see in my life? You have to be totally honest with yourself—also to get to the bottom of the causes of your weight "without blinders." Pure, "bare" self-reflection is the keyword for starting (as you know from Chap. 3). Sustainable weight loss requires:

- a healthy body with a functioning metabolism,
- strong willpower,
- perseverance,
- resilient self-confidence,
- psychological and physical stress/tolerance of deprivation, and
- a lot of effort (maybe even calorie counting).

4.4 Modern Apps Meet Old-School Tool

If you still want to count kilocalories, or continue to do so, but don't want to do everything by hand or in your head, there are modern tech tools: Many people find that a calorie-counting app or a calorie calculator on their smartphone or PC helps with weight loss. Take your time to thoroughly research whether and which of these IT support options might suit you. With this little digital helper, many people seriously, consciously, and focusedly engage with their own eating and dietary habits for the first time in their lives. In addition, many apps can also scan, evaluate, and manage foods. This makes it quick and easy to learn and document how many calories are in particular products and portions. For example, if you like to snack on a "small" 150-g can of cashews or peanuts while binge-watching in the evening, you'll be surprised to read: You've just consumed a hefty 1000 kcal. And often just as a side note—because it's so salty, often washed down with plenty of liquid calorie bombs like beer, wine, or cola. Besides calorie counting, it's just as important to know: How much of what am I actually allowed to eat?

In addition to the app, a kitchen scale is essential—because knowing how many kilocalories are in 100 g is one thing, but knowing how much you actually eat or drink is another; this is also crucial to avoid exceeding your target calorie amount.

This is, at its core, the essence of any diet—and now you know it. But what else matters? You may remember: The diet has to suit you—and only you know best what really suits you.

Therefore, only foods that you enjoy eating, that you like, that taste good to you, and that you tolerate well should be at the center.

You don't need to worry if you don't meet the supposed "healthy" eating guidelines like "eat fruit and vegetables five times a day." That doesn't matter—you'll find out why in Chaps. 16 and 17. If you want to lose weight in the long term and avoid the yo-yo effect—and that is exactly the goal of this book and your journey to your new slim self—then you should choose a diet that suits you in the long term, that you enjoy, that brings you joy, and that you can and, above all, want to maintain forever. What you should aim for is therefore much more than a diet; it is a kind of fundamental, permanent dietary change that becomes a new attitude toward life. Therefore, the term "diet" will rarely be mentioned from now on when it comes to your personal "weight loss project."

4.5 Dietary Change Becomes a New Attitude Toward Life

In the sober language of medical professionals, it currently sounds like this: “The goal of effective nutritional therapy is to adjust the diet so that food intake with a daily energy deficit of 500 kcal per day can be achieved … The key factors for the chosen dietary strategy (for weight reduction) are consideration of individual eating and dietary habits as well as food preferences and wishes of the patients (with obesity). ‘The goals, principles, and practical aspects of dietary change should be explained, and the individual dietary recommendations should take into account the personal and professional environment. These aspects are crucial to promote high short- and especially long-term compliance’ (Becker and Zipfel 2020).

Find the range of your individual negative energy balance in which you can achieve **maximum weight loss with minimal deprivation** in the long term.

4.6 Humans Are Not Machines

Even if 500 kcal below requirements may seem moderate—for the body, too little is simply too little to “maintain” itself. It must and will, therefore, adjust its metabolism during the “weight reduction process” when it truly comes down to the body’s own substance: Basal metabolic rate and heat production are gradually and subtly reduced, sometimes noticeably so: You feel cold more easily, less capable, and become tired more quickly.

"The body adapts over the course of a diet. In a sense, it learns to make better use of the changed food supply and to extract more from less food. "The effect is that at some point, you stop losing weight or may even gain weight again, even though you are eating less and differently than before," explains Prof. Arved Weimann, obesity expert and chief physician, Klinikum St. Georg, Leipzig (Tenzer 2021).

This, in turn, means that the simple rule of three for continuous weight loss may apply for a while, but then, due to the body's own metabolic adaptation, weight loss can stagnate: Weight loss stalls, you lose fewer kilos than expected, or perhaps nothing happens on the scale for a while. You need to be aware of this. Otherwise, the "human machine calculation" would look like this: If a deficit of 500 kcal per day leads to a weight loss of 2 kg per month, you would lose 24 kg in a year—almost 50 kg in two years; and eventually, you would "disappear." Our bodies cannot continuously lose the same amount of weight indefinitely with an identical negative energy balance. Therefore, the organism must adjust its metabolism—and this is achieved by the aforementioned reduction in energy expenditure.

Therefore, the following can happen: If you consume only 1500 kcal per day instead of 2000 kcal, your body may, after a certain amount of weight loss and adaptation, also lower its basal metabolic rate accordingly. Then, perhaps, not much will happen on the scale anymore. This biological-energetic adaptation protection mechanism can also lead to you regaining weight more quickly if you increase your daily calorie intake again. How long the body maintains this process of reduced basal metabolic rate and decreased heat production is neither generally known nor can a valid statement be made for an individual. In any case, the body continues this for a while after a diet—hence the well-known yo-yo effect; especially pronounced after crash diets and rapid weight loss. Therefore, think and plan slowly and for the long term, otherwise you will not achieve lasting success. Also, be prepared for "setbacks." So, change your eating habits moderately and sustainably to your new dietary style with plenty of patience and time—and observe your body closely. This makes success most likely, but still does not guarantee it within the planned timeframe. Because: There is no universal recipe here. Everyone must find their own individual path. The aforementioned principle also applies to a negative energy balance: There is no one perfect calorie deficit for everyone, as each body reacts individually to a permanent energy shortage depending on its condition and metabolism. Some trial and error may be necessary until you find your optimal calorie deficit that "works" (= weight loss) and allows you to live well. For this reason, take a little more time to get to know yourself, your body, and its adaptation mechanisms in different phases—and how to deal with them in harmony with body and mind, so that you continue to feel good and remain satisfied. It is your very own "journey to your new desired weight."

4.7 Don't Forbid Anything! Don't Put Yourself Under Pressure!

Let's briefly recap the basics: When it comes to losing weight, the core principle is to consume fewer calories than you burn. You can eat anything you like. The only thing that needs to be reduced is the portion size and the total amount. One more essential point:

> If you enjoy something, you should "include it in your plan" and eat it. Otherwise, you'll create a craving—which will find its way "out" in uncontrolled overeating.

Regardless of your personal preferences, it is generally advisable to eat something from each of the three macronutrients—carbohydrates, fat, and protein—so that the meal is not only enjoyable but also nutritionally balanced. In particular:

> Don't skimp on protein—it's not only an important building block for body tissue such as muscles, but protein also keeps you feeling full for a particularly long time.

This trilogy of energy/building blocks is not only more satisfyingly filling for the body, but also for the taste buds in your mouth and nose—and thus for your psyche. Good keyword: Don't put your psyche under pressure with unrealistic goals, stay stress-free. This helps enormously in making your journey to your desired weight a relaxed one. Even if it takes a little longer—it's worth it. And now …

… your journey to a slimmer you can begin.

Caution: Alcohol!

One important tip must not be missed: When calculating your energy balance, don't "forget" or underestimate alcohol! Pure alcohol contains 7 kcal per gram—that's almost as much as 1 g of fat (9 kcal). Alcohol therefore provides more energy than protein and carbohydrates (4 kcal per gram). Anyone wanting to lose weight should know this—and take it into account, i.e., plan for it and include it in calculations.

Just one 0.75-liter bottle of dry red wine with 14% alcohol easily adds up to about 700 kcal—or better said: to your hips. If, after that, the physiologically activated craving for something savory kicks in—who doesn't know this after a boisterous evening—and you treat yourself to a good half a bag of chips (not even the whole bag), your adipocytes (your fat cells) will be delighted with another 500 kcal … Together, that's almost the daily requirement of a strict reduction diet. So, be strict with yourself during the day if you plan to indulge in the evening and still want to stay in a calorie deficit. But beware: Alcohol on an almost empty stomach quickly goes to your head—the "pathway to the brain" is clear …

In addition: Anyone who drinks (a lot of) alcohol significantly inhibits their fat burning. The reason: Even though we drink alcohol because we enjoy it and it's fun—the body immediately recognizes alcohol as a dangerous, toxic substance whose breakdown is extremely important. Therefore, the liver eliminates the toxin alcohol immediately. Conversely, fat metabolism slows down—which means less body fat is broken down. And, just to remind you again so you don't forget: Alcohol also makes you hungry—anyone who has ever been out partying will remember that special moment at the end of the night when there's only one need left: "I need something really hearty and tasty to eat now!" Even die-hard vegetarians can be tempted. A British vegetarian survey found: More than a third eat meat when they're drunk—and their favorite is kebab!

Conclusion: Regularly high alcohol consumption, due to the triple mechanism of "less fat burning + more eating + alcohol calories," can not only lead to the infamous beer belly in the long term, but also to overall weight gain. As always, however: It's the total energy balance that counts.

For some people who like to drink a lot, the only "master key to weight loss success" may be: Just consistently cut out alcohol for a while. If you see yourself in this description, you're done reading, can get started, and dry out your fat stores. But you'll surely still be interested in what else is important for sustainable weight loss …

Important Note

The range of individual weight loss in diet studies is always very large: Some participants lose a lot of weight very quickly, others extremely slowly and very little. If, despite a clearly negative energy balance, you lose very little or nothing in the short to medium term, it is best to have your doctor check whether you may have a disease, metabolic disorder, and/or fat distribution disorder.

Key Points of the Chapter

The fundamental basic recommendations to start your weight loss:

- Before making a long-term dietary change to lose weight, you must be clear about:
  - Why am I/why do I feel overweight, where did/do the unwanted kilos come from?
  - What is my goal? Where do I want to go and why?
- The new way of eating must suit the person—not the other way around. Therefore:
- Everyone should choose only the hypocaloric (= energy-deficient) diet that is individually ideal for: character, lifestyle, daily routine, metabolism, chronobiology, preferences, and dislikes.
- The dietary change must be lived in harmony and close connection with body and mind, and should not be seen or used as a "weapon" against oneself.
- Eat only what you like, what tastes good, does you good, and agrees with you. You do not need to be "afraid" of unhealthy foods (see Chaps. 16 and 17).
- Eat a varied and diverse diet with fresh, high-quality foods.
- Explicitly allow yourself to enjoy—consciously celebrate these moments of pleasure in peace, with all your senses, and above all: relaxed and stress-free.
- Make sure to eat at least one truly enjoyable, satisfying meal each day.
- Avoid "snacks"/nibbles between meals as much as possible (keyword: keep insulin levels low).
- With (almost) calorie-free drinks and foods, you have a "flatrate"—eat and drink as much and as often as you like.
- Sustainable weight loss with long-term maintenance of the new, reduced weight requires: time, perseverance, attention, patience.
- So do not plan for just the next four weeks or months, but: years. Losing weight is not a sprint, but a long-distance run—it takes work and can be exhausting.

- Therefore, "diet" is basically the wrong term; better is: "Long-term/permanent dietary and lifestyle change that fits me, my work, and family life."
- The master key, the universal key to weight loss, is a negative energy balance: consume fewer calories than you expend.
- A healthy/physiologically acceptable calorie deficit for moderate weight loss is considered to be 500 kcal below requirements per day.
- So if you use about 2000 kcal/day, your "energy-reduced diet" for initial weight loss is 1500 kcal per day. For a short period (a few days), you can reduce to as little as 1200 kcal if necessary.
- The key to sticking with it is the right balance—find your individual daily calorie intake: it must be balanced so that you can tolerate the "energy deficit" well and still lose weight as desired.
- Whether you primarily reduce carbohydrates or fats or both does not matter.
- It is best not to reduce protein (good for satiety, important for muscle maintenance/building).
- Actual weight loss is about 2–2.5 kg per month.
- As a general target, a weight loss of 5–10% of body weight per year is recommended.
- Choose a fixed weigh-in day per week, that's enough. Weighing yourself every day is pointless, only causes stress, and makes you nervous.
- Stay calm and relaxed. Be generous and kind to yourself if things do not go as planned; setbacks and periods of stagnation will always occur.
- Aiming for a new, lower weight that makes you feel better is also an act of self-care, which should be experienced with joy and fun.
- Mindset reflection, relaxation, and physical activity (more on this later) are important companions to a long-term successful dietary change that leads to your new desired weight for good.

4.8 Summary: Your Current Level of Knowledge

At this point on your journey to your new desired weight, you now know…

- All diets are based on the same principle: negative energy balance.
- There is no better or worse diet—all diets are the same.

- Most weight loss programs fail and lead to weight gain because they are both impersonal and not tailored to the individual, and are only carried out for a short time.
- The result: the vicious circle/circulus vitiosus:
  (new) diet fails ➔ weight gain ➔ fear of failure/self-doubt ➔ (new) diet fails ➔ …
- Classic diets are therefore considered a "gateway drug" to eating disorders and obesity.
- Trendy diets such as low carb and intermittent fasting are also no better than other diets, no matter what the media, influencers, and celebrities write and post.
- My new path begins with honest self-awareness: I must be clear about who I am and what I want. My mindset must align with this. Then I can get started.
- **Sustainable slimming/weight loss is basically simple at first: With a moderate energy deficit of about 500 kcal per day, you lose about 2 kg per month.**
- **Find the range of your individual negative energy balance in which you achieve the perfect personal balance between maximum weight loss and minimal deprivation in the long term.**
- **How you achieve this negative energy balance is up to you—it depends on your eating preferences and lifestyle. Essential: The dietary change must suit you, your body, and your daily life; you must feel comfortable with it.**

References

Becker S, Zipfel S (2020) Verhaltenstherapie bei Adipositas. Cardiovasc 20(3):35–41

Tenzer E (2021) Der Speck bleibt weg. Apotheken-Umschau A/01/2021, S 48–52

test (2021) Intervallfasten. Seltener essen – aber wie? https://www.test.de/Intervallfasten-Seltener-essen-aber-wie-5451361-0/?mc=news.2021.01-01-Intervallfastenundm_i=6BJ1RaF8MJYBnQTjyqt3V9053Ks7WcSpbEFb-zB5S9O8GCOV78MrPwMzIm3VSBtX0gVe2MmLu2MBFoQaK38EC9I-So3PxV1M. Accessed: 4. Jan. 2020

AWMF (2024) S3-Leitlinie Prävention und Therapie der Adipositas. https://register.awmf.org/de/leitlinien/detail/050-001. Accessed: 3. März 2025

Knop U (2024) Adipositas-Leitlinie 2024. Abnehmen leicht gemacht – so klappt's mit der individuellen Ernährung. https://www.focus.de/gesundheit/abnehmen-leicht-gemacht-so-klappt-s-mit-der-individuellen-ernaehrung_id_260492113.html. Accessed: 3. März 2025

test (2023) Diätkonzepte im Test: Welche Diät beim Abnehmen hilft https://www.test.de/Diaetkonzepte-im-Test-Welche-Diaet-beim-Abnehmen-hilft-6072458-0/. Accessed: 3. März 2025

5 Staying Slim—The "Secret" of Maintaining Weight

"You can't stay on a diet forever."

This wisdom is now common knowledge. And you should not—and do not have to—"stay on a diet forever." Failure would be inevitable. What you are planning—redundancy is intentional here, as it is essential—is not a diet in the classic sense, which starts and then ends. With your mindset shift, there is no "after the diet" period. Rather: This is about a permanent change in both your diet and your entire lifestyle. This may proceed more relaxed and achieve visible desired results more slowly, but these results are sustainable. The underlying "secret," which is gradually gaining recognition, is revealed as follows:

> Firmly and permanently implement your new lean lifestyle at the core of your life.

Your main goal is also clear: to maintain the weight you have reduced with much effort, exertion, and sacrifice at your desired level in the long term. How do I do that? That is the quintessential "Gretchen question."

U. Knop, *Successful and Sustainable Weight Loss*,
https://doi.org/10.1007/978-3-662-72477-4_5

And the answer is: It is a lifelong task, often anything but easy—but not necessarily so. Because those in the minority with a mindset vein that continues to pulse actively, and who have managed to maintain their reduced weight long-term, have one thing in common: They simply stayed consistent and committed. They maintained what they had switched to their new mindset during their initial weight loss phase—in a moderately modified form. But they continue to live by and with their new lifestyle—because they like it and because they do not want to fall back into their "weight-gaining loops." And that is ultimately all there is to it. As banal as it may sound: You have to want not to fall back into old patterns. You have to prefer the way you live now. And it is precisely with this premise in mind that you should plan and approach your sustainable lifestyle change. There is neither a "blueprint" nor valid data from research, because:

"In the past, nutritional medicine has mainly focused on how overweight people can best lose kilos, and has hardly developed any concepts for how to maintain weight afterwards," laments Prof. Stephan Bischoff from the Institute of Nutritional Medicine at the University of Hohenheim (Schumacher 2021).

This revelation regarding "no general plan for weight maintenance" is not just an individual opinion, but is now also echoed clearly in medical journals, which therefore also focus on the individual approach:

"Long-term weight loss represents the greatest challenge in the treatment of overweight and obesity ... The previous ineffectiveness of interventions for health-promoting behavior change ... may be due to insufficient consideration of individual characteristics ... and can be explained by the fact that recommendations for restrictive eating behavior [author's note: for example, calorie counting, energy and quantity reduction] probably cannot be generalized, but would have to change depending on the individual situation and in the process of long-term weight loss ..." (Neumann and de Zwaan 2020)

5.1 Focus on a Feel-Good Life

So it remains your individual challenge in the sense of I DIET MY WAY. The new small number on the scale, at which you truly beam inside, is important as a core metric, no question. But at least as relevant for long-term success is that you feel really comfortable with your new weight and can maintain it permanently, without your life turning into constant ascetic self-mortification. This will only succeed for the rest of your life if your meals still truly taste delicious and satisfy you at the same time. This will not be the case with every meal. But that should be your aim. Because constant hunger makes it much harder to stick to the new lifestyle.

If you have lost weight and become significantly lighter, you no longer need to consume as much energy as before your body transformation to meet the basic needs of your reduced weight. Therefore, special attention should be paid to your own post-diet weight development, observing how your "new" body now reacts to different calorie intakes.

Have you reached your feel-good weight? Now the task is to maintain this "neobody" in the long term by simply continuing your new life. Simple—it sounds so easy, and in principle, it is. In practice, this means: Stay on your successful path and stick to your new habits. Be aware: There is no ideal weight for everyone—every person eats and is different.

5.2 Don't "Leave Behind" Relaxation and Exercise

Don't forget to take your good (new) achievements in terms of relaxation and exercise with you into your new life (more on this in Chap. 7). These two cornerstones should also be firmly anchored in your new lifestyle. In particular, the body's powerhouses must continue to be nurtured and cared for, because: With regular exercise and (over)exertion, your muscle cells grow. And the larger they are and become, the more energy the body consumes, even at rest, when doing nothing. This "function" not only makes losing weight itself easier, but also helps maintain the new body weight:

> "Physical training plays a crucial role, especially in preventing renewed weight gain, that is, in the weight stabilization phase after successful weight loss." (Becker and Zipfel 2020)

In this context, a very large study (Paixão et al. 2020) is of significant practical relevance: This "systematic review" aimed to answer the following question: "Which strategies promise the greatest success in preventing weight regain after a diet?" To this end, Portuguese university scientists examined the findings of five different national weight control registries (from Germany, Portugal, Finland, Greece, and the USA)—and for the first time: "To our knowledge, this is the first systematic review of information on successful weight loss obtained from weight control registries." In their comprehensive review, the researchers summarized the results from 52 studies published by the aforementioned weight control registries. A brief note: These national weight control registries document and analyze findings on what specifically can help prevent weight regain after a diet—in other words, how to maintain weight. Now, the exciting question: What results did the researchers publish?

People who not only successfully lost weight but also maintained their weight loss in the long term cited some dietary strategies such as increased consumption of vegetables and reduced intake of foods high in sugar and fat. But—among all strategies, increased physical activity was the key factor most consistently associated with "maintaining reduced weight." The researchers summarized their key finding as follows:

> "Increased physical activity was the most consistent positive correlate of weight loss maintenance." (Paixão et al. 2020)

Although this is only a correlate (i.e., a statistical association, see Chap. 16) and it is therefore not certain what causal influence increased physical activity has on weight maintenance, it is still interesting to know: Physical activity "unites" those who have remained slim … that should be a weighty argument to pay attention to it. Perhaps it will work for you as well. Another common marker of all long-term successful weight maintainers is "the higher level of restrictive eating behavior" (Neumann and de Zwaan 2020)—this also seems plausible, because those who no longer pay attention to conscious food choices, calorie counting, energy, and quantity reduction quickly fall back into old patterns and weight classes.

5.3 Long-Term Weight Stabilization

The two aforementioned authors, Becker and Zipfel, sum it up nicely in their paper—even though it concerns obese patients in the doctor's office, at its core, everyone who wants to lose weight goes through the same pattern with the same pitfalls and identical solution strategies: "The common problem of weight reduction programs lies less in achieving short-term weight loss and more in stabilizing the weight loss achieved … Permanent behavior change can occur when new habits are established in patients' everyday lives. This only works if the methods for lifestyle change regarding diet and physical activity learned in the basic program (for weight reduction) are repeated over and over until they subsequently become automated … Here, the focus is on practicing behaviors aimed at improving health, satisfaction with what has been achieved, and no longer on further weight loss."

5.4 Health!

Health, a good keyword—because nowadays, this is the new "therapeutic target" for the medical community, even when it comes to weight reduction. The primary goal is no longer to achieve the supposed ideal weight according to BMI (Body Mass Index), in other words, to "lose weight at all costs"—but rather to reach a completely individual weight that leads to maximum health and greater well-being. "The treatment of overweight should focus on improving health and well-being, not just on weight loss," is roughly the current consensus of the Canadian guideline (Wharton et al. 2020). Here, too, a paradigm shift toward a holistic view of the human being is emerging. A welcome development.

Key Points of the Chapter

- There is no "big secret" to staying slim.
- You can only sustainably maintain your weight at your desired and comfort level by permanently changing and maintaining your new eating habits.
- Other lifestyle factors that help maintain a healthy weight, such as physical activity and relaxation, are also beneficial (see Chap. 7).
- In particular, increased physical activity is what "unites" those who have successfully maintained weight loss in the long term.
- Therefore, the key to "eternal slimness" is: Maintain your new healthy lifestyle habits, stay committed, and continue on your successful path.
- The right mindset, your new attitude—"Mindset is the game changer."
- Be kind and honest with yourself, have patience, and forgive yourself for mistakes.
- Enjoy your personal development and the increased self-confidence you have developed in harmonious alignment with your body.
- It's not about "that one number" on the scale, but about a holistic, healthy sense of overall well-being.
- Ultimately, it's not about losing as much weight as possible in a few weeks or months, but about sticking with it for life—and consciously increasing your quality of life.
- It is essential not to "forget" enjoyment, as it is also holistically important—researchers at the University of Zurich showed in a study: "People who can fully indulge in enjoyment not only experience greater well-being in the short term, but also have higher overall life satisfaction and, among other things, experience fewer symptoms of depression and anxiety" (Bernecker and Becker 2020).

5.5 Summary: Your Current Level of Knowledge

At this point on your journey to your new desired weight, you now know…

- All diets are based on the same principle: negative energy balance.
- There is no better or worse diet—all diets are the same.
- Most weight loss programs fail and lead to weight gain because they are both impersonal, not tailored to the individual, and only carried out for a short period.
- The result: the vicious cycle/circulus vitiosus:
  (new) diet fails ➔ weight gain ➔ fear of failure/self-doubt ➔ (new) diet fails ➔ …
- Classic diets are therefore considered a "gateway drug" to eating disorders and obesity.
- Trendy diets like low carb and intermittent fasting are also no better than other diets, no matter what the media, influencers, and celebrities write and post.
- My new path begins with honest self-awareness: I need to be clear about who I am and what I want. My mindset must align with this. Then I can get started.
- Sustainable weight loss is basically simple at first: With a moderate energy deficit of about 500 kcal per day, you lose about 2 kg per month.
- Find the range of your individual negative energy balance in which you can achieve the perfect personal balance between maximum weight loss and minimal deprivation in the long term.
- How you achieve this negative energy balance is up to you—it depends on your food preferences and your lifestyle. Essential: The dietary change must suit you, your body, and your daily life; you must feel comfortable with it.

- **The "secret key" to staying slim is: Keep going and stay committed. Maintain your dietary and lifestyle changes. Your "diet" (which never really was one) becomes your new lifestyle, which you ideally maintain forever—simply because you feel so good with it!**

References

Becker S, Zipfel S (2020) Verhaltenstherapie bei Adipositas. CARDIOVASC 20(3):35–41

Bernecker K, Becker B (2020) Beyond self-control: mechanisms of hedonic goal pursuit and its relevance for well-being. Personal Soc Psychol Bull. https://doi.org/10.1177/0146167220941998

Neumann M, de Zwaan M (2020) Restriktives Essverhalten und langfristige Gewichtsabnahme. Adipositas Ursachen Folgeerkrankungen Therapie 14(02):107–113

Paixão et al (2020) Successful weight loss maintenance: a systematic review of weight control registries. Obesity Rev. https://doi.org/10.1111/obr.13003

Schumacher B (2021) Schlank ohne Jo-Jo-Effekt: Wie Sie Ihr Gewicht halten. https://www.oekotest.de/gesundheit-medikamente/Schlank-ohne-Jo-Jo-Effekt-Wie-Sie-Ihr-Gewicht-halten-_107323_1.html. Accessed: 10. Jan. 2021

Wharton et al (2020) Obesity in adults: a clinical practice guideline. CMAJ 192(31):E875–E891. https://doi.org/10.1503/cmaj.191707

6

I DIET MY WAY!

"A diet should be adapted to individual preferences so that the way of eating can continue to be enjoyable. In addition, a successful diet must be practical in everyday life and tailored to one's life situation. And it has to taste good, because otherwise, failure is usually inevitable." (BMEL 2020)

With this beautiful, worth-reading "state statement" from the Federal Ministry of Food, we begin the central chapter. But first, please recap briefly: Would you have thought that the "science of losing weight" is basically as simple as described in the previous chapters? With more than 500 diets, all of which claim the "holy grail of eternal slimness" exclusively for themselves, it seems somewhat paradoxical that at their core, they are all the same. Old wine in new, trendy bottles. But, as you now know, it's all about marketing: diet providers have to position themselves as the current best slimming solution, one that, as a sales bonus, "celebrities swear by." And for that, a USP is needed. In sales jargon, this is the acronym for Unique Selling Point—which means "the uniqueness, the special feature that sets a product apart from the competition in a positive way." Therefore, diet providers invent an "emotionally soothing cloud" of outstanding features around the ever-same

U. Knop, *Successful and Sustainable Weight Loss*,
https://doi.org/10.1007/978-3-662-72477-4_6

negative energy balance, designed to convey a pleasant sense of superiority: losing weight with little or no carbohydrates, eating low-fat, vegetarian, meals only at certain times, counting points, analyzing blood and genes, and many more clever inventions to boost sales—because every year a new diet trend is needed, since the previous ones, as usual, did not lead to the desired success. You don't need any of that (anymore); you can now laugh about it and ignore the trends. Now it's about you, about your very own, individually created path to your new desired slim weight: I DIET MY WAY!

6.1 You Decide, No One Else

Some of the "essence of knowledge" about diets that follows is already fundamentally familiar to you from the previous chapters. In the following, you should once again engage fully, both emotionally and self-reflectively, with the path you choose for yourself and want to follow—take some time to ponder and philosophize about which paths will be yours and which will not. The following questions require your answers:

- What is my goal?
- By when do I want to achieve what?
- How much energy have I consumed daily so far?
- What have I eaten and drunk, and why?
- How do I achieve a negative energy balance of about 500 kcal below my needs?
- How do I reduce my calorie intake to (1200 to) 1500 kcal per day?
- What do I eat and drink on my journey, what do I leave out?
- Do I use a calorie app and/or do I document by hand in my "weight loss diary"?
- What else is important to me?

You need to be clear about what your weight loss, your new slim self, is "worth" to you—which sacrifices you expect and are willing to make for your goal. You also know the risks: eating disorders, yo-yo effect, weight gain with more body fat, bad mood... all of this may await you on your journey. It may, but it doesn't have to. That is why it is essential that you make your path as wonderful as possible.

6.2 Tabula Rasa First

The foundation of the intended long-term dietary change is: First, make a clean slate. So, analyze your current nutritional status quo. For this, you can either use a classic food diary, in which you accurately record everything you eat and drink for two to three weeks. Alternatively, you can use an app on your smartphone—which saves time and effort, especially for those who are tech-savvy. In addition, many of these calorie-tracking apps already have numerous foods pre-installed, including their calories, nutrient content, etc. Afterwards, you will have an overview of your total energy intake up to now. Now you can tackle your targeted calorie deficit—at the beginning, if possible, do not exceed the modest "minus 500 kcal" and try it with a maximum of 1500 kcal per day. This way, you can approach the change in your diet moderately.

6.3 Negative Energy Balance

Even if you might be tired of hearing it, the negative energy balance is the be-all and end-all, the foundation of weight reduction. But even the "minus 500 kcal" to lose weight sustainably and comfortably is, of course, only a guideline. If you notice that with 1500 kcal per day (i.e., 500 below the average consumption of a woman with 2000 kcal), not much is happening on the scale, then try the following:

> In the meantime, reduce—slowly and carefully—in small steps down to a minimum of 1200 kcal per day.

You should not go lower, as this value is considered the likely "threshold for metabolic shift"—which means that less than 1200 kcal comes close to a crash diet, and your body very quickly switches to "starvation survival mode," drastically slowing down your metabolism, basal metabolic rate, and heat production. You don't want that, as it greatly undermines long-term success; the likelihood of yo-yo effect and the like increases rapidly. But you see: you have a bit of individual "energy leeway," even downward, if you wish. However, the very low calorie amount of 1200 kcal should not be maintained for too long, as this increases the likelihood of hunger attacks, metabolic derailments, and last but not least, failure. A few consecutive days should be sufficient at the beginning if you are aiming for this lower limit for the first time.

6.4 The Culinary Celebration Highlight

Once you have decided which individual strategy for dietary change you want to use to lose weight, feel free to follow this little insider tip: Integrate—a "culinary celebration highlight" into your daily routine, within your personal calorie limit. A delicious culinary treat that you really enjoy eating. A piece of your favorite chocolate or a special cake, particular chips or gummy bears, or something savory that you "love on your tongue." The amount doesn't matter; on the contrary, less is more. What matters is this: Enjoy it with all your senses, with full focus, and celebrate eating it slowly—mindful, timeless enjoyment is the key to the culinary "bullet-time moment." This slow-motion enjoyment is yours, and yours alone. Treat yourself to it, even every day if you like.

6.5 Ensure Quality and Variety on Your Plate

The basic rule is: Since you will be eating less and choosing more carefully, you should prefer fresh, high-quality foods—because good food of high quality often tastes better as well. Above all, try out new foods and meals that are less "energy-dense" than your usual favorites. This means the dishes provide fewer calories for the same amount and volume. Research the term "energy density principle" online—it's fascinating to see that meals that look almost identical can deliver only half as many calories. That can be an advantage. Scientifically, a comprehensive meta-analysis (of 13 individual publications) by researchers at the German Institute of Human Nutrition (DifE) has also shown: "In summary, our study provides further evidence supporting the energy density of foods as a simple but effective measure for weight control in overweight individuals aiming for weight reduction" (Stelmach-Mardas et al. 2016). Or more simply: By consuming foods with low energy density, body weight can be reduced in overweight (obese) individuals.

For example: A crispy breaded Wiener schnitzel with golden fried French fries and a hearty, thick mushroom sauce easily delivers twice the energy of a "plain" peppered schnitzel with oven-baked rosemary potato wedges and tomato-oregano sauce. Or: Instead of a double-cheese salami pizza with 900 kcal, simply try a version that provides only 600 kcal. Maybe it tastes just as good and you feel just as full. With burgers, spaghetti, potato casseroles, and basically everything, you can and should experiment and vary by gradually lowering the calories per weight. Just test where your personal lower limit of satiety lies with different meals. You might notice, for example, that you already feel full at breakfast with 300 kcal instead of the usual 500, if you eat two slices of bread with a little cheese and ham, but with more fresh "calorie-free crunchy toppings" like tomato, cucumber, and lettuce, instead of heavily loaded baguettes. As an "energy principle," the following applies: Wherever and whenever possible, reduce calorie-rich sides like pasta, potatoes, or rice, and simply eat more vegetables or salad—in fact, cauliflower, broccoli, cucumbers, tomatoes, and cabbage provide almost zero calories with plenty of volume. Of course, only if they are not drowned in rich fatty sauces. Admittedly, the feeling of fullness achieved by high volume and low energy is not very sustainable or long-lasting, but it helps to curb hunger in the moment—and perhaps to realize in general: "Oh, interesting, that really is enough."

> You can drink and eat as much as you like of drinks and foods that are "free from" calories at any time.

As always, the important thing is: There are no forbidden foods on your plate, your cutting board, or in your hand—there are also no unhealthy foods or any obligation to stick to a "healthy diet" (Chaps. 16 and 17 explain why). You try and create what you want to eat—the relevant point is and remains: It must taste really delicious to you, you must tolerate it well, and not feel "stuffed to the brim" afterwards. Be creative with your culinary innovations!

6.6 Mastering the Pitfalls of Everyday Life

Anyone who has ever wanted to lose weight or has already tried knows it well: The biggest hurdles are those that everyday life itself presents and provides. And there are plenty of them. Temptations here, invitations there, cravings and a guilty conscience as companions, the fear of falling back into old, "excessive" eating habits, and the worry that the "bad" excess weight will return—and that you might fall into the yo-yo trap again. The occasional "Now it doesn't matter anyway" thought-demon can also easily dominate your actions. People who have felt overweight all their lives also say: "The feeling of being fat doesn't go away so quickly." You have to deal with that too and keep "mind(re)setting" yourself—even if the fear of gaining weight again doesn't let go of you, be aware of what you want: for example, to continue feeling relaxed when you look in the mirror, because you like what you see, because you (now again) like your reflection and accept yourself as you are (or have become).

6.7 No Vacation—A Lifelong Journey Over Years (or Decades)

What you should also know: To lose weight sustainably and permanently, it takes more than a diet for a short period: What is required is a long-term change in eating habits that you ideally maintain forever—because it suits you, brings you joy, culinary satisfaction, and the knowledge that you are preserving your newly slimmed figure. Because one of the core problems is: After the diet, many people go back to eating as they did before. A relapse into old unhealthy fattening patterns is not uncommon—with the well-known rebound effect: the kilos come back. And you don't want that either. It is therefore essential to remain patient. So, gladly give yourself and your body the time you and it need—gradual is the key, stay realistic, and celebrate milestones and small successes. This way, you maintain the basic motivation for a long-term change in diet at a high level. Another important message is: Even if you don't succeed in losing weight permanently and keeping it off on your first try, admit the failure, let go of the past, and try again. Just try a different plan that fits your lifestyle (even) better. Regardless, you can of course change your nutrition plan at any time if you want to, because you feel the need or simply want to vary things—you are the "head chef in the ring." Just dare to do whatever you like.

6.8 Eat Until You Are Full!

This subheading may sound a bit paradoxical when it comes to losing weight, but it is completely free of mockery and irony. Because eating until you are full is also essential for long-term success. Enjoying a feeling of fullness gives the body peace and satisfaction. Of course, you can't enjoy this all the time, because your overall energy balance still needs to be negative. But—and this is important—at the few meals you "have available," you should eat until you are full. That just means there are fewer calories left for the rest of the day. Or there were fewer before, and you eat your fill in the evening. Whether at lunch, in the morning, or whenever—that depends on your chronobiology (that is, your day-night rhythm and when your body gets hungry), your preferences, and your lifestyle. In any case, the following should apply:

> Once a day, eat until you are enjoyably full!

A weight loss program in the sense of a sustainable change in diet will only be successful in the long term if the meals are truly satisfying—even if only for a short time, but the feeling must be real and authentic. Not only the calorie and/or fat content (fat = most intense flavor carrier) or protein content (= satiety factor) of the foods and/or meal play an essential role: The amount and volume also have a direct, immediate influence on the perception of genuine satiety. When the stomach is well filled, a pleasant feeling of fullness can also develop.

6.9 Sleep Well!

One aspect that should be explicitly mentioned here is the core relevance of the "dark side" of our lives—namely, the night, when we sleep. Healthy sleep is the foundation for a healthy life. Numerous studies over the past decades have observed the correlation: the poorer the quality of sleep and the shorter the night's rest, the higher the risk of overweight and obesity. Even though—as is always the case with correlations (more on this in Chap. 16)—we can only speculate about cause and effect and a potential causality, a simple appeal to common sense suffices: Those who sleep too little and too poorly will, sooner or later, certainly do their health no favors and may even develop lasting problems. Therefore, especially in the new phase of dietary change, lifestyle modification, and weight reduction—which is certainly physically and mentally demanding at first—maintaining healthy "sleep hygiene" is essential. Make sure you sleep well and long enough.

In this context, an interesting new study (Wickham et al. 2020) examined which of the three fundamental lifestyle factors—sleep, nutrition, or activity—is most important for mental health. You can probably guess the result:

> Sufficient restorative sleep is the most important pillar of mental health; in the study, good sleep was the strongest predictor (predictive factor) for mental health and well-being.

Surprisingly for the researchers, sleep quality was more important than duration. Ergo, it can be clearly stated here as well: quality over quantity. And you should, of course, apply this credo to your dietary change as well: eat less, but eat better.

6.10 The Central Chapter

You decide how you want to lose weight, how quickly, with what methods, and over what period of time. It is important to focus on the following values:

- Your own self-determination,
- Responsibility,
- and sovereignty of decision.

Successful weight loss only works if you follow your very own path with self-respect and self-love—I DIET MY WAY!

If the ever-recurring mantra of this chapter title reminds you of a song—you are right. Music enthusiasts, please be "gracious" now: A verse from the legendary song by Frank Sinatra, whose title inspired the name for this approach to achieving your desired weight, is, by chance, also quite relevant to the content of this book:

> Yes, there were times, I'm sure you knew
> When I bit off more than I could chew
> And through it all, whenever there was doubt
> I ate it up and spit it out
> I faced it all and I stood tall
> And did it, did it my way

Translated into German:

> Ja, es gab Zeiten, ich bin sicher, Du wusstest es
> Wenn ich mehr abgebissen habe, als ich kauen konnte
> Und das alles, wann immer es Zweifel gab

Ich habe es gegessen und ausgespuckt
Ich habe alles durchgestanden und stand aufrecht
Und – I DIET MY WAY!

With a – admittedly – broad potential for free-spirited interpretation, one could perfectly transfer this verse to the topic of diets and nutrition:

In the past, there were times when I ate far too much,
far beyond my hunger –
and especially in phases of life when I wasn't doing so well,
when I had doubts about myself and my life,
it was so much that I overate and had to throw up.
But in the end, I stood tall and true to myself
and said: I will follow the diet that suits me best,
I will follow my own path of nutrition.

Well then—certainly such an abstract "cover song" in a book about sustainable weight loss is not everyone's cup of tea. But it could become your "hit of success." Because whenever you stand in front of the mirror (as you will), to enjoy your new, thoroughly slimmed-down silhouette, you will know: I owe this success entirely to myself, to my strength and perseverance, to my resilience in the face of setbacks, and to my iron will to follow my path and stay on it. And when you take pleasure in yourself, just sing or hum "I DIET MY WAY …" and enjoy the positive effect of this beautiful melody!

The Most Important Points of the Chapter

- The era of "losing weight according to external plans" or even "off-the-shelf diets" is over.
- I DIET MY WAY means: Only those who reshape their lives on their own initiative with far-reaching lifestyle adaptations—so that the new path fully fits their own personality—will succeed in sustainable weight loss.
- Anyone who wants to become slimmer should create and follow their very own path to long-term weight reduction—and stay on it for life.

6.11 Summary: Your Current Level of Knowledge

At this point on your journey to your new desired weight, you now know…

- All diets are based on the same principle: negative energy balance.
- There is no better or worse diet—all diets are equal.
- Most weight loss programs fail and lead to weight gain because they are both impersonal and not tailored to the individual, and are only carried out for a short period.
- The result: the vicious circle/circulus vitiosus:
  (new) diet fails ➔ weight gain ➔ fear of failure/self-doubt ➔ (new) diet fails ➔ …
- Classic diets are therefore considered a "gateway drug" to eating disorders and obesity.
- Trendy diets like low carb and intermittent fasting are no better than other diets, no matter what the media, influencers, and celebrities write and post.
- My new path begins with honest self-awareness: I must be clear about who I am and what I want. My mindset must align with this. Then I can get started.
- Sustainable slimming/weight loss is basically simple at first: With a moderate energy deficit of about 500 kcal per day, you lose about 2 kg per month.
- Find the range of your individual negative energy balance in which you achieve the perfect personal balance between maximum weight loss and minimal deprivation in the long term.
- How you achieve this negative energy balance is entirely up to you; it depends on your eating preferences and your lifestyle. Essential: The dietary change must suit you, your body, and your daily life; you must feel comfortable with it.
- The "secret key" to staying slim is: keep going and stick with it. Maintain your dietary and lifestyle changes. Your "diet" (which never

really was one) becomes your new lifestyle, which you ideally maintain forever—simply because you feel so good with it!

- **I DIET MY WAY means: You decide which path you want to take—and you should stay on that path. You can adapt it at any time to your current wishes and needs—or even completely "tailor" it new if a change in lifestyle requires it. You are the boss in your own ring!**

References

Bundesministerium für Ernährung und Landwirtschaft (BMEL) (2020) Gesundes Abnehmen. https://www.in-form.de/wissen/gesundes-abnehmen/. Accessed: 28. Dez. 2020

Stelmach-Mardas et al (2016) Link between food energy density and body weight changes in obese adults. Nutrients 8(4):229. https://doi.org/10.3390/nu8040229

Wickham et al (2020) The big three health behaviors and mental health and well-being among young adults: a cross-sectional investigation of sleep, exercise, and diet. Front Psychol. https://doi.org/10.3389/fpsyg.2020.579205

7 Ideal Support: Relaxation and Exercise

The two ideal companions to a diet—defined here as a "long-term, lifelong, individualized change in eating habits to maintain the newly achieved desired weight permanently"—are: on the one hand, relaxation exercises for mental strengthening and psychological reinforcement of your plan, and on the other hand, physical activity/sports to boost energy expenditure, stimulate circulation, and maintain and "keep in operation" muscle mass. In short: mind and body stay in the flow.

7.1 Relaxation: Yoga & More

Let's start with "mental support." Whether you enjoy meditating, prefer autogenic training or progressive muscle relaxation, love practicing yoga, or whatever else you choose, that is entirely up to you—even if you don't feel like doing anything for "soul relaxation," that is absolutely fine. The credo of this book applies here as well, the common thread: voluntariness and honesty. Only integrate relaxing activities into your life that you genuinely want to do, out of your own free will, from "intrinsic motivation" (from within), and be honest with yourself about

U. Knop, *Successful and Sustainable Weight Loss*,
https://doi.org/10.1007/978-3-662-72477-4_7

it. You want to do it. You feel like doing it. Only then will relaxation exercises for unwinding and "winding down" truly bring you positive benefits in life.

Below you will find some yoga exercises that can help you not only to relax and critically reflect on your I DIET MY WAY project, but also to stimulate your metabolism. These are tried-and-true yoga poses that have been successfully practiced by many people for a long time.

Selected Yoga Exercises

- Downward-Facing Dog
- Warrior 1 and 2
- Seated Twist
- Heart-opening backbends such as Cobra or Upward-Facing Dog

The most important aspect of all exercises should always be conscious breathing: deep inhalation down to below the navel and complete exhalation starting from the same spot. For everything else, if you are interested, you will need to read up in the relevant books or websites—and then get started. Just give it a try and see if yoga is good for you.

7.2 Sports: Get Moving!

The following section on physical activity is a bit more extensive. It doesn't always have to be sports. There is no single "royal road" that works for everyone and leads everyone to their goal. Physical activity is fundamental—there's no need to debate that. Someone who only sits, lies down a lot, and barely moves will, sooner or later, find their body, circulation, and metabolism lacking in "somatic momentum." Therefore, the motto is: Move your body. The key questions are:

- Which type of activity or sport, at what frequency and intensity, is best for whom at which stage of life?
- What brings the greatest benefit for body and mind?
- What is good for whom, and why?

The answer is as simple as it is individual: only you can find that out for yourself. Only the type of sport that truly brings you joy and genuinely good feelings, that you approach with inner motivation—only those activities are the best and right ones for you. Therefore, you will not find a recommendation here along the lines of "This or that sport is the ultimate, do this and skip that"—instead, you will get an overview of the factors that are fundamentally important for finding the sport that suits you. Before that, and that's why this chapter exists in this book, you will learn why physical activity and sports are important building blocks of a successful "slimming down" project and how integrative bodywork can contribute to long-term weight loss.

7.3 Muscles—the Turbocharger for Basal Metabolic Rate

With a sustainable change in diet, the main goal is long-term weight loss. That is: not just to become slim, but above all to stay slim. Another important building block is the permanent preservation of muscle mass—or even better, if new muscles can be built during the weight loss process. Why? It's simple: muscles are the body's power plants, responsible for a high basal metabolic rate. In other words: the more muscle you have, the higher your energy expenditure even at rest—and this accounts for an estimated 70–80% of total energy expenditure. For this reason, it is essential that muscles do not "melt away" during weight loss—which is why it's called losing fat, not "losing muscle." This undesirable side effect of weight reduction can't be completely avoided—but, and this is the good news, you can actively counteract diet-related muscle loss. And you should: with exercise, especially strength training. That's why sports—or let's say muscle movement training—are so important in the process of active weight loss. There's also the aesthetic aspect: a muscular, well-trained body often looks better, both to oneself and to others, than flabby, soft body parts with a strong tendency toward gravity. Although, of course, that is a matter of personal perspective and should not be made into a dogma. Beauty is always in the eye of the beholder.

Keep your muscles moving—and promote their growth!

So, what are the two main reasons why physical activity and athletic training should be considered as permanent companions in weight loss? At their core, it's simple: maintain a high basal metabolic rate and preserve body tension. Building muscle mass helps both women and men to boost their own metabolism. Those who "own" more muscle mass simply burn more energy, even while sitting, lying down, or sleeping. In addition—if you enjoy what you do—physical activity can also have a positive effect on your mental well-being. In general, it can be said: any kind of movement and physical activity stimulates the metabolism and increases energy expenditure—both of which are very beneficial for long-term weight loss success. What activities you choose is entirely up to you.

7.4 Movement Must Be Fun!

The decisive factor is the "joy of doing." And: being active regularly. Whether you are a jogger, walker, spinner, swimmer, biker, HIIT enthusiast (High-Intensity Interval Training), or whatever else—it doesn't matter, as long as you enjoy it. Or do you prefer "real sports" like tennis, soccer, table tennis, handball, or squash? Then do that. For many, having an activity partner is the right "complementary element." Training together can not only be more fun, but also increases commitment, you motivate each other—and the inner couch potato has to convince not only you but also your workout partner. Training with your own body weight is especially recommended for solo exercisers, as you don't need a gym, no equipment, no worries about getting there or parking, and your schedule is flexible. This type of training is also called "bodyweight exercise" (BWE)—you use only your own body weight and almost completely forgo aids like weights and fitness machines. Calisthenics is particularly popular here. In this outdoor variant, various pull-up bars, parallel bars, and monkey bars are available in workout parks, where you train using your own body weight. But that's more for advanced practitioners, where your own belly doesn't get in the way during push-ups …

7.5 Grab Some Dumbbells!

If you're still unsure which "physical exercise" is right for you, here's a simple tip: get some dumbbells and lift them. Dumbbells make it easy to get started—you can pick up the "steel" anytime and train with it. The dumbbells are always there for you—because in terms of location, timing, and duration, you literally have everything in your own hands. Whether you do a few exercises of your choice for 5–10 minutes in the morning before work, in the evening, or whenever—it will do your muscles good, keep them active, and depending on the weight, you'll build muscle particularly quickly (especially for "dumbbell novices" who have never trained before, strenuous strength training can lead to rapid, visible muscle growth). If iron and steel are your workout of choice, get informed—it's quick to learn. As simple basic rules, remember: the higher the weight and the lower the maximum possible repetitions (i.e., the number of dumbbell lifts, about 5 to a maximum of 10), the faster your body builds new muscle. Conversely: the lower the weight and the more often you repeat the exercise, the more the training strengthens your existing muscles, their definition, and endurance. In short: there's something for everyone with dumbbells—anyone can lift them.

7.6 The Right Mix Matters!

Another important principle in sports is: create synergies. In the "premier league," you combine several types of sports with different focuses, that is, strength and endurance training in intervals: one week with weights, one week of cardio training, or something different every day.

Ideally, combine endurance training with strength training.

Important: None of this is meant as a specific recommendation for you personally, but is simply intended to objectively and professionally convey the current state of science regarding the "ideal sport." Because one thing is clear: with a little bit of "working out," you will not lose significant weight. That requires intensive training: One hour on the treadmill, cross trainer, stepper, rowing machine, or jogging outdoors burns about 800–900 kcal. One hour! That is not insignificant. Especially if done regularly, twice a week or more. So, the main point here and now is not to turn you into an athlete, but to actively support your weight-reducing dietary adaptation, to gradually improve your overall physical fitness, and above all, not to feel compelled to be fit and look good, but rather: to feel good while doing it! To benefit from this feel-good effect of exercise, you do not need a sophisticated training plan. Doing it—that's what matters.

7.7 More Movement in Everyday Life!

However, if you really have no desire for sports, you should consciously focus on your daily movements. Every day offers a wide range of diverse options to move more. Even if the following tips are surely familiar, here they are again as a reminder.

Tips for more movement in everyday life

- Take the stairs instead of the elevator—occasionally two steps at a time
- Use your lunch break for a "power walk" or simply go for a stroll
- Schedule movement breaks at the office: stand up and do a few loosening exercises
- Increase your housework and gardening workload—very efficient and inexhaustible
- Do daily errands on foot or by bike instead of by car
- Just go for a walk in the fresh air "for no reason" and clear your head, air out your brain

If you take a moment to sit down and calmly review your days in detail in your mind's eye, you will surely uncover even more opportunities in your daily routine to incorporate more movement—beyond the standard tips mentioned above. There is also something new to report from research, because not only does your body benefit from daily movement while losing weight, but your psyche does too: "Everyday activities also increase well-being," announced a press release from the Karlsruhe Institute of Technology and the Central Institute of Mental Health in Mannheim on the occasion of their new study (Fodi 2020). "Physical activity makes you happy and is important for maintaining mental health. The results show that even everyday activities like climbing stairs have a significant benefit for well-being." Physical activity significantly improves physical well-being and mental health. The researchers examined how everyday activities such as climbing stairs, walking, or running to catch the tram affected the participants' well-being. They found that immediately after everyday activity, participants felt more alert and energized. "Alertness and energy, in turn, were demonstrably important components of the well-being and mental health of the study participants," the scientists concluded.

It is important for you to know regarding movement: It is never too late to start. And you should stick with it. And above all, not only when it comes to eating but also with exercise: Always listen to your body's signals. If it does not feel like exercising and needs rest, you should allow yourself that break—and not push through at all costs. Otherwise, you will quickly give up when your body "shuts down." In this sense: Always act in a balanced way. Have fun!

And finally, a rhythmic movement tip—if you really have no desire for anything sporty: Dance!

Put on your favorite music and dance—following the holistic flow of your body, to the beat of your inner rhythm. With this individual dance style, your whole body and mind are set in motion. A quarter of an hour of living room dancing every day—anyone who has tried it knows not only how pleasantly sweaty but also how wonderfully liberating it can be. If your surroundings allow and you can sing loudly while doing it—even better, because that doubles the fun and relieves stress.

It is also important not to place too much hope in the effect of "working out" when it comes to losing weight, because: "It should be noted that exercise therapy alone does not achieve significant and clinically relevant weight reduction, but only the combination with reduced calorie intake is successful" (Becker and Zipfel 2020). Something else is much more realistic and relevant: So let us conclude "officially" and let the Federal Ministry of Food and Agriculture comment on "exercise as a weight loss booster": "What matters is that movement is fun, because that is the best reason to stick with it" (BMEL 2020).

The Most Important Points of the Chapter

- Regular relaxation and movement are the best support duo for a long-term successful dietary change to sustainably reduce weight.
- Combine endurance training with strength training plus everyday activities.
- Only do the type of exercise that you personally (most) enjoy.
- The point is that you feel good doing it.
- The best "basal metabolic turbo booster" is muscle—make sure to maintain and build it: Get some dumbbells and lift steel.
- Increase and intensify your movements in everyday life.
- See movement and relaxation as the supportive yin & yang that will permanently accompany your successful dietary change.

7.8 Summary: Your Current State of Knowledge

At this point in your journey toward your desired new weight, you now know ….

- All diets are based on the same principle: a negative energy balance.
- There is no better or worse diet—all diets are the same.
- Most weight loss programs fail and actually lead to weight gain, as they are both impersonal, not tailored to the individual, and only implemented for a short period of time.
- The result: the vicious circle/circulus vitiosus:

(new) diet fails ➔ weight gain ➔ fear of failure/self-doubt ➔ (new) diet fails ➔ …

- Classic diets are therefore considered a "gateway drug" to eating disorders and obesity.
- Trendy diets like low carb and intermittent fasting are no better than other diets, no matter what the media, influencers, and celebrities write and post.
- My new path begins with honest self-awareness: I need to be clear about who I am and what I want. My mindset must align with this. Then I can get started.
- Sustainable weight loss is basically simple at first: With a moderate energy deficit of about 500 kcal per day, you will lose around 2 kg per month.
- Find the range of your individual negative energy balance in which you can achieve the perfect personal balance between maximum weight loss and minimal sacrifice in the long term.
- How you achieve this negative energy balance is entirely up to you—it depends on your eating preferences and your lifestyle. Essential: The dietary change must suit you, your body, and your daily life; you need to feel comfortable with it.
- The "secret key" to staying slim is: keep going and stick with it. Maintain your dietary and lifestyle changes. Your "diet" (which never really was one) becomes your new lifestyle, which you ideally maintain forever—simply because you feel so good with it!
- I DIET MY WAY means: You decide which path you want to take—and you should stick to it. You can adapt it at any time to your current wishes and needs—or even completely "tailor" it anew if a change in lifestyle requires it. You are the boss in your own ring!
- **Make sure to include targeted phases and oases of relaxation and self-reflection. Continually update your mindset to the "latest version of yourself."**
- **Keep moving. It doesn't have to be "real hard-core sports." Choose the activities that you truly enjoy again and again. Freestyle dancing at home is a real option.**
- **Keep your muscles active with dumbbells.**

- **And don't forget: The more (new) movements you permanently integrate into your daily routine, the better for the long-term, sustainable overall success of the project.**

References

Becker S, Zipfel S (2020) Verhaltenstherapie bei Adipositas. CARDIOVASC 20(3):35–41

Bundesministerium für Ernährung und Landwirtschaft (BMEL) (2020) Gesundes Abnehmen. https://www.in-form.de/wissen/gesundes-abnehmen/. Accessed: 28. Dez. 2020

Fodi S (2020) Forschungsergebnisse – Auch Alltagsaktivitäten steigern das Wohlbefinden. https://nachrichten.idw-online.de/2020/11/19/auch-alltagsaktivitaeten-steigern-das-wohlbefinden/. Accessed: 26. Dez. 2020

8

SWOT Yourself!

You have now reached the point where you slowly but surely know everything you need to make a decision: Should I change my diet and choose I DIET MY WAY?! To make this perhaps still difficult (and weighty) decision easier for you, you should now conduct a double SWOT analysis of yourself and your project "Losing Weight."

SWOT what? The SWOT analysis is a basic tool in marketing used to evaluate a product or service in four dimensions. In a matrix, the four dimensions—Strengths (S for "strengths"), Weaknesses (W for "weaknesses"), Opportunities (O for "opportunities"), and Threats (T for "threats")—are compared. And that is exactly what you should now do holistically for your planned dietary change—because afterwards, you will know yourself and your plan even better, be able to reflect more deeply, and last but not least, make this fundamental decision based on additional important facts and factors. Do not limit your SWOT analysis only to your dietary adaptation for weight loss, but also include yourself, your personality, your own characteristics—and other lifestyle factors you want or plan to change.

U. Knop, *Successful and Sustainable Weight Loss*,
https://doi.org/10.1007/978-3-662-72477-4_8

As a little "jump start," here are some possible answers for each of the four categories—some of which you will surely remember from previous chapters.

Strengths (S)

- Perseverance (me)
- Willpower (me)
- Exactly my taste (dietary change [D])
- Meets my needs (D)

Weaknesses (W)

- Residual hunger remains (D)
- Counting calories is "annoying" and error-prone (D)
- Willpower is not enough (me)
- Uncertainty about whether I can do it (me)

Opportunities (O)

- Dream weight! (me)
- More satisfaction and quality of life (me)
- Permanent dietary change that I enjoy (D)
- Switch to a healthier eating style (D)

Threats (T)

- Project fails—yo-yo effect—weight gain (D)
- Muscle loss and eating disorders (D)
- Depressed mood/self-doubt due to failure (me)
- Dissatisfaction with myself/the situation (me)

With the above examples, you can now go "in medias res" with yourself and your project. Here, too, the universal credo that runs like a red

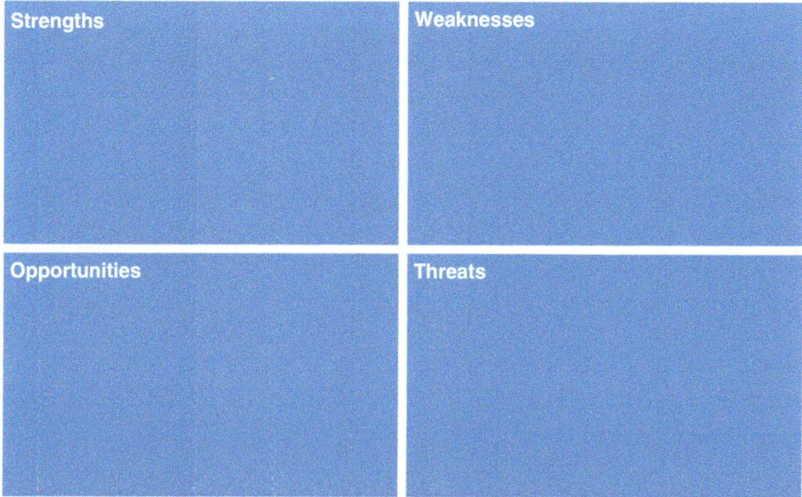

Fig. 8.1 SWOT Analysis ME

thread through the entire content of the book applies: Be honest, leave nothing out, and do not "sugarcoat" the truths and your realities. This is about you and your future. So now—enjoy and gain (hopefully surprising) insights as you conduct your individual SWOT analysis!

Now create a double **SWOT analysis**—both of yourself and of your "Losing Weight" project. Figures 8.1 and 8.2 serve as templates, which you can copy or fill in directly here in the book with your own ideas.

Key Points of the Chapter

- Before you get started, you should be clear not only about your strengths and weaknesses, but also about the opportunities and threats, and analyze them (SWOT).
- It is best to do this SWOT analysis in two versions: for yourself—your self, your personality—and for your dietary change for weight reduction.

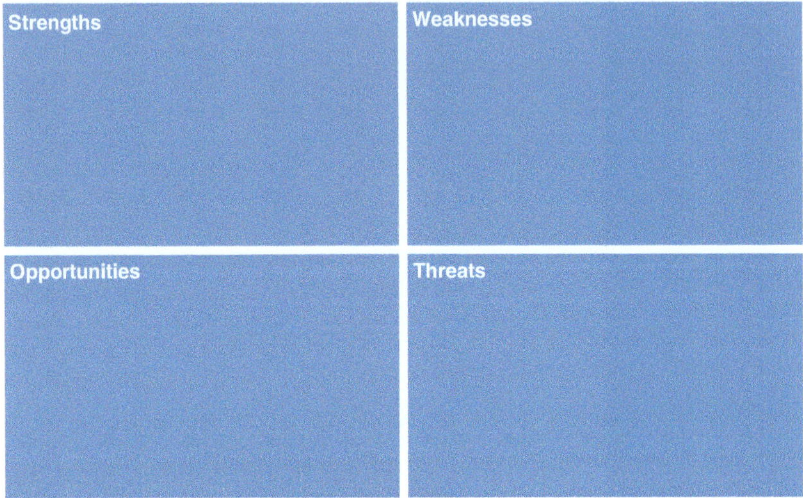

Fig. 8.2 SWOT Analysis DIETARY CHANGE

8.1 Summary: Your Current State of Knowledge

At this point in your journey toward your desired new weight, you now know ….

- All diets are based on the same principle: a negative energy balance.
- There is no better or worse diet—all diets are the same.
- Most weight loss programs fail and actually lead to weight gain, as they are both impersonal, not tailored to the individual, and only carried out for a short period of time.
- The result: the vicious circle/circulus vitiosus:
  (new) diet fails ➔ weight gain ➔ fear of failure/self-doubt ➔ (new) diet fails ➔ …
- Classic diets are therefore considered a "gateway drug" to eating disorders and obesity.

- Trendy diets like low carb and intermittent fasting are no better than other diets, no matter what the media, influencers, and celebrities write and post.
- My new path begins with honest self-reflection: I need to be clear about who I am and what I want. My mindset must align with this. Then I can get started.
- Sustainable weight loss is basically simple at first: With a moderate energy deficit of about 500 kcal per day, you will lose around 2 kg per month.
- Find the range of your individual negative energy balance in which you can achieve the perfect personal balance between maximum weight loss and minimal sacrifice in the long term.
- How you achieve this negative energy balance is entirely up to you; it depends on your eating preferences and your lifestyle. Essential: The dietary change must suit you, your body, and your daily routine—you need to feel comfortable with it.
- The "secret key" to staying slim is: keep going and stick with it. Maintain your dietary and lifestyle changes. Your "diet" (which never really was one) becomes your new lifestyle, which you ideally maintain forever—simply because you feel so good with it!
- I DIET MY WAY means: You decide which path you want to take—and you should stick to that path. You can adapt it at any time to your current wishes and needs—or even completely "tailor" it anew if a change in lifestyle requires it. You are the boss in your own ring!
- Make sure to include targeted phases and oases of relaxation and self-reflection. Continually update your mindset to the "latest version of yourself."
- Keep moving. It doesn't have to be "real hard-core sports." Choose the activities that you truly enjoy again and again. Freestyle dancing at home is a real option.
- Keep your muscles active with dumbbells.
- And don't forget: The more (new) movements you permanently integrate into your daily life, the better for the long-term, sustainable overall success of the project.
- **Do a double SWOT analysis—both of yourself and of your "getting slimmer" project.**

9

The 16 Success Factors and Your Wish List

What makes a long-term, sustainably successful dietary change for weight reduction? In theory, it's quite simple—you know the most important factors. The following list now shows the essential criteria in detail. Regularly check your own "DIET WAY" to see whether all or at least most of the factors that match your new mindset are still being met. Afterwards, you'll find a small "wish list" that you can fill out not only for yourself. Feel free to send your answers for anonymous evaluation to the author of this book: uwe.knop@gmail.com

The 16 Success Factors

A long-term successful dietary change for sustainable weight reduction is characterized by the following: It must...

1. ...fit me, my life(style), and my "budget",
2. ...be based on my chronobiology,
3. ...take my intuitive eating preferences into account, i.e., always allow free choice from all foods,
4. ...only "provide" foods, dishes, and drinks that I enjoy eating, that taste good to me, and that I tolerate well,

U. Knop, *Successful and Sustainable Weight Loss*,
https://doi.org/10.1007/978-3-662-72477-4_9

5. ...offer pleasure and make me feel "truly satisfied" at least once a day,
6. ...allow a culinary delight/a gourmet highlight each day,
7. ...avoid total bans and restrictions,
8. ...prevent cravings so that they do not arise in the first place,
9. ...give me the freedom to always act/adapt flexibly and spontaneously,
10. ...always be adaptable in the long term if changes in my lifestyle require it,
11. ...be easy for me to implement on my own, without necessarily needing a "coach",
12. ...make me happy and satisfied—I enjoy doing it!—,
13. ...provide me with all the necessary nutrients I need for a healthy life,
14. ...actually lead to a sustainable dietary change that I am happy to maintain for life,
15. ...achieve the goals I have set for myself,
16. ...lead to the desired weight loss and make me slimmer—permanently!

Take the points listed above in hand from time to time and compare them with your own long-term dietary change. Because you, and only you, have it in your hands to ensure that your lifestyle adaptations also become your desired way of eating—you decide how to proceed. If you see that many of the criteria are not being met: Reflect on why that is—and whether you want to do something to achieve the outstanding points in the future. This should definitely be done if you are dissatisfied with yourself, your eating behavior, and your body or weight.

9.1 Your Personal Top 3

Now we come to the previously announced, very personal "What else do I wish for?" list. What is especially important to you when losing weight, beyond the basics mentioned above? For example, "I want to stay muscular" or "My sexual drive/libido must not decrease, let alone be 'switched off'" or "My joy in life should remain the same or grow" or "I absolutely do not want to lose weight from my breasts" or "The dietary change should also convince my circle of friends to join in" or "Finally find the love of my life" or "Become attractive to men/women" or "Not be stared at reproachfully when eating in a (fast food) restaurant" or "Finally shop in designer stores that carry my size" or "The feeling should disappear that people are laughing and gossiping about me behind my back" or … Here is space for everything you wish for. Listen deep inside yourself, be honest, and don't be ashamed of anything—no one but you needs to know, but: *You* need to know. The better you know yourself and your inner wishes, your very own instinctive needs, and honestly reflect on them, the better! Because the more you know about yourself and are aware of what you really want and what you don't, the better you can tailor your "weight loss" project to your own personality—and the greater your chances of achieving what you set out to do. Dare to, be brave—and let's get started:

My personal top 3 wishes/requirements for a long-term dietary change for sustainable weight reduction are:

1. ______________________________
2. ______________________________
3. ______________________________

The same applies here: Try to make sure that your wishes and reality match. But don't be disappointed if one of the requirements cannot be implemented or realized—because you know: Life is not a wish concert. What matters is that, in the end, you feel better and have a higher quality of life! In this spirit, let's turn to the next chapter, where you will set your goal achievement plan. Because that, too, is important for success: Visualize your goals, fix them, and on the way there, critically and constructively check how real life matches the goals you have set. The journey is the goal. That's right, because it will probably be a lifelong project—one that should and ideally will "give" you joy and satisfaction. But the (milestone) goals are along the way. Achieve what you set out to do. For yourself. For your ego. For your well-being. For the inner affirmation "Yes, I want it, I can do it, I will do it, I will succeed—and I will stick with it!" And of course, the following also applies: Flexibility and "wish adaptation" according to your lifestyle are always possible. You decide.

The Most Important Points of the Chapter

- Check your "slimming" project for congruence/alignment with the fundamental 16 success factors—try to achieve as many of them as possible.
- Write down your three most important personal "additional wishes" for your project—and become clear about why you want to achieve these top 3 in particular.

9.2 Summary: Your Current State Of Knowledge

At this point in your journey toward your desired new weight, you now know …

- All diets are based on the same principle: a negative energy balance.
- There is no better or worse diet—all diets are the same.
- Most weight loss programs fail and actually lead to weight gain, as they are both impersonal, not tailored to the individual, and only carried out for a short period of time.
- The result: the vicious circle/circulus vitiosus:
  (new) diet fails → weight gain → fear of failure/self-doubt → (new) diet fails → …
- Classic diets are therefore considered a "gateway drug" to eating disorders and obesity.
- Trendy diets like low carb and intermittent fasting are no better than other diets, no matter what the media, influencers, and celebrities write and post.
- My new path begins with honest self-awareness: I need to be clear about who I am and what I want. My mindset must align with this. Then I can get started.

- Sustainable weight loss is basically simple at first: With a moderate energy deficit of about 500 kcal per day, you will lose about 2 kg per month.
- Find the range of your individual negative energy balance in which you can achieve the perfect personal balance between maximum weight loss and minimal sacrifice in the long term.
- How you achieve this negative energy balance is entirely up to you—it depends on your eating preferences and your lifestyle. Essential: The dietary change must suit you, your body, and your daily life; you must feel comfortable with it.
- The "secret key" to staying slim is: keep going and stick with it. Maintain your dietary and lifestyle changes. Your "diet" (which never really was one) becomes your new lifestyle, which you ideally maintain forever—simply because you feel so good with it!
- I DIET MY WAY means: You decide which path you want to take—and you should stay on that path. You can adapt it at any time to your current wishes and needs—or even completely "tailor" it anew if a change in lifestyle requires it. You are the boss in your own ring!
- Make sure to include targeted phases and oases of relaxation and self-reflection. Continually update your mindset to the "latest version of yourself."
- Keep moving. It doesn't have to be "real hard exercise." Choose the activities that you truly enjoy again and again. Freestyle dancing at home is a real option.
- Keep your muscles active with dumbbells.
- And don't forget: The more (new) movements you permanently integrate into your daily routine, the better for the long-term, sustainable overall success of the project.
- Do a double SWOT analysis—both of yourself and of your "getting slimmer" project.
- **Check: How close is your project to the ideal version? Also reflect and document: What else do I expect, what is still personally important to me?**

10

Nutrition-, Enjoyment-, and Feelings-Diary

A food diary is generally recommended as an established "tool" for successfully implementing dietary changes—helping to develop, in the medium to long term, a heightened awareness for more mindful eating habits. What do I eat, when, how often—and why, actually? Often, this is the first time one fully reflects on and then analyzes their own diet. This process can reveal some surprises, such as, "Aha, I wasn't even aware of how much I unconsciously consume on the side in a week…"

To ensure your personal insights provide immediate added value, Table 10.1 serves not only as a food diary, but also as a pleasure and feelings journal. The purpose is not to add up the calories consumed—a smartphone app or a PC calorie calculator can do that better. Here, the focus is on the "meta-view of the bigger picture"—see what insights about yourself you can gain after one or two weeks.

U. Knop, *Successful and Sustainable Weight Loss*,
https://doi.org/10.1007/978-3-662-72477-4_10

Table 10.1 My food, pleasure, and feelings diary

	Monday	Tuesday	Wednesday	Thursday	Friday	Saturday	Sunday
How many times did you eat today?	• 1× • 2× • 3× • 4× • 5× • >5×	• 1× • 2× • 3× • 4× • 5× • >5×	• 1× • 2× • 3× • 4× • 5× • >5×	• 1× • 2× • 3× • 4× • 5× • >5×	• 1× • 2× • 3× • 4× • 5× • >5×	• 1× • 2× • 3× • 4× • 5× • >5×	• 1× • 2× • 3× • 4× • 5× • >5×
Did you eat mainly because you were truly hungry?	• yes • no • not sure	• yes • no • not sure	• yes • no • not sure	• yes • no • not sure	• yes • no • not sure	• yes • no • not sure	• yes • no • not sure
How did you feel after meals/snacks? Mostly …	• very good • good • so-so • not so good • bad	• very good • good • so-so • not so good • bad	• very good • good • so-so • not so good • bad	• very good • good • so-so • not so good • bad	• very good • good • so-so • not so good • bad	• very good • good • so-so • not so good • bad	• very good • good • so-so • not so good • bad
Which food/snack was the pleasure highlight of the day?							
And what was the opposite, that is, the "culinary turn-off"?							
How satisfied were you today with your eating behavior?	• very • normal • so-so • not at all	• very • normal • so-so • not at all	• very • normal • so-so • not at all	• very • normal • so-so • not at all	• very • normal • so-so • not at all	• very • normal • so-so • not at all	• very • normal • so-so • not at all

(continued)

Table 10.1 (continued)

	Monday	Tuesday	Wednesday	Thursday	Friday	Saturday	Sunday
How hungry were you when you went to bed today?	• very • clearly noticeable • a little • not at all	• very • clearly noticeable • a little • not at all	• very • clearly noticeable • a little • not at all	• very • clearly noticeable • a little • not at all	• very • clearly noticeable • a little • not at all	• very • clearly noticeable • a little • not at all	• very • clearly noticeable • a little • not at all
How many kcal did you consume today? (Use calorie calculator)							
Did you lose weight today?	• yes • no • not checked	• yes • no • not checked	• yes • no • not checked	• yes • no • not checked	• yes • no • not checked	• yes • no • not checked	• yes • no • not checked
How satisfied are you with your weight development this week?	"	"	"	"	"	"	• very • so-so • not at all

10.1 Two-to-Three-Week Report: Eating & Drinking

In addition, you should also record everything you eat and drink, and when, for two to three weeks as accurately as possible—remember: please do not deceive yourself. Be as honest as always, even if true self-reflection can sometimes be painful… You are doing this to learn from it, to develop better eating habits, and to lead a more enjoyable life.

It is best to create this documentation **before** you start your lifestyle and dietary changes—simply to recognize what, when, why, and in what quantities you eat and drink. So, write down exactly what you have eaten and drunk every day. You can do this in the "traditional" way, by handwriting it in a notebook in your own style—and then use an app or an online calorie calculator to roughly sum up how many kilocalories you have "assimilated" per day. Or you can analyze everything fully digitally right from the start. There are numerous programs that make this easier: just search the internet or app store for "calorie calculator, diary, or counter." From these two weeks, you can already derive initial calorie amounts that you will need to save in the future—according to your personal plan. Also note when and why you eat (out of hunger or non-hungry emotional eating due to stress, habit, frustration, sorrow, boredom). This way, you can honestly reflect again and consider if and where/when there is definitely potential for savings. This insight can be helpful in tailoring your dietary changes. For example, if you realize that you absolutely need to include chocolate in your food choices and reserve calories for it every day—then do so. Or you find that you definitely need to eat a hot meal in the evening and that this meal should not be skipped—keyword biorhythm/chronobiology, i.e., are you a natural early or late eater, do you have more real, physical hunger in the morning or evening? This is often anchored in your genetics, in your chronobiological genes. You will be able to answer these and other questions for yourself—and in doing so, you will get to know yourself even better, so you can tailor your project plan in detail to your own personality.

Key Points of the Chapter

- Keep a food diary that also serves as a pleasure and mood journal.
- Document your eating & drinking habits in detail for 14 days **before** starting the project.
- Analyze openly and honestly what you have learned about yourself in your two "self-reflection documents."

10.2 Summary: Your Current State of Knowledge

At this point in your journey toward your desired new weight, you now know ….

- All diets are based on the same principle: a negative energy balance.
- There is no better or worse diet—all diets are the same.
- Most weight loss programs fail and actually lead to weight gain, as they are both impersonal, not tailored to the individual, and only carried out for a short period of time.
- The result: the vicious circle/circulus vitiosus:
  (new) diet fails ➔ weight gain ➔ fear of failure/self-doubt ➔ (new) diet fails ➔ …
- Classic diets are therefore considered a "gateway drug" to eating disorders and obesity.
- Trendy diets like low carb and intermittent fasting are no better than other diets, no matter what the media, influencers, and celebrities write and post.
- My new path begins with honest self-awareness: I need to be clear about who I am and what I want. My mindset must align with this. Then I can get started.
- Sustainable weight loss is basically simple at first: With a moderate energy deficit of about 500 kcal per day, you will lose about 2 kg per month.

- Find the range of your individual negative energy balance in which you can achieve the perfect personal balance between maximum weight loss and minimal sacrifice in the long term.
- How you achieve this negative energy balance is up to you—it depends on your eating preferences and your lifestyle. Essential: The dietary change must suit you, your body, and your daily life; you must feel comfortable with it.
- The "secret key" to staying slim is: keep going and stick with it. Maintain your dietary and lifestyle changes. Your "diet" (which never really was one) becomes your new lifestyle, which you ideally maintain forever—simply because you feel so good with it!
- I DIET MY WAY means: You decide which path you want to take—and you should stick to that path. You can adapt it at any time to your current wishes and needs—or even completely "tailor" it anew if a change in lifestyle requires it. You are the boss in your own ring!
- Make sure to include targeted phases and oases of relaxation and self-reflection. Continually update your mindset to the "latest version of yourself."
- Keep moving. It doesn't have to be "real hard-core sports." Choose the activities that you truly enjoy again and again. Freestyle dancing at home is a real option.
- Keep your muscles active with dumbbells.
- And don't forget: The more (new) movements you permanently integrate into your daily routine, the better for the long-term, sustainable overall success of the project.
- Do a double SWOT analysis—both of yourself and of your "getting slimmer" project.
- Check: How close is your project to the ideal version? Also reflect on and document: What else do I expect, what is still personally important to me?
- **Keep an "Eat & Feel Diary."**
- **Before starting the project, document your current eating and drinking habits for 14 days.**

11

My Master Plan to Reach My Goal

If you know what you want, the path to get there becomes easier—because you also know *where* you want to go. Therefore, create a "master plan" for achieving your goals—with intermediate milestones, at which you should reward yourself when you reach them. Don't be too strict or overly ambitious with your "target values," as this only creates unnecessary pressure—and leads to frustration or disappointment if you "fail."

You have all the time in the world, because what you are planning is a lifelong task—and not an easy one, but a demanding challenge. So allow yourself enough flexibility—you can always adjust your goals upward if you find you are progressing faster than planned. This way, the entire "project of becoming slimmer" is much more enjoyable, as you can approach it more relaxed and will be able to celebrate successes.

Consider the following goal achievement criteria as initial inspiration to formulate your own personal goals. At the end, visualize the "final goal" in your mind's eye: How do you see yourself, what do you want to see, how do you want to look? But first, formulate your concrete goals (Table 11.1).

U. Knop, *Successful and Sustainable Weight Loss*,
https://doi.org/10.1007/978-3-662-72477-4_11

Table 11.1 My master plan for my new target weight

Start date of my long-term dietary change to achieve lasting weight loss:
Starting weight:
Fat mass (if you have such a scale):
Waist circumference:
Clothing size shirts/tops:
Clothing size pants/bottoms:
Skin changes: sagging/fat aprons (personal perception on a scale of 1–10/1 = very poor/10 = excellent, wonderful)
Psychological factors: satisfaction, self-love, feeling more attractive and valuable (scale 1–10/1 = very poor/10 = excellent, wonderful)
My other personal goals:

Enter your other very personal goals in the last column, for example: that and when you will be able to wear your "favorite pants from the recent past" again—because they finally fit you again. Or: more muscle mass in the chest, shoulders, legs, upper arms, specified in centimeters. Or tying your shoes without getting red-faced and out of breath. For example, the well-known TV chef Frank Rosin lost 18 kg permanently with his "long-term dietary change." When asked, "How has this changed your body awareness?" he replied: "I simply feel better and much healthier. It's a great feeling to look down at myself and be able to say again: That's how it's done" (BMEL 2019).

In this spirit, let your thoughts run free! (Tables 11.2 and 11.3)

Table 11.2 After 6 months I want to achieve:

Weight:
Fat mass:
Waist circumference:
Clothing size shirts/tops:
Clothing size pants/bottoms:
Skin changes; sagging/fat aprons:
Psychological factors:
Other personal goals:

Table 11.3 After 12 months I want to achieve:

Weight:
Fat mass:
Waist circumference:
Clothing size shirts/tops:
Clothing size pants/bottoms:
Skin changes; sagging/fat aprons:
Psychological factors:
Other personal goals:

11.1 And My Final Goal Looks Like This

Forever, for life, I want to …

11.2 Use Your Imagination!

Finally, a small "dose of autosuggestion": Close your eyes—and now visualize in your mind's eye how you see yourself once you have achieved your desired goal. What do you see? What do you feel when you imagine this sight? You probably like it a lot, right? Then stick with it! Action—that's the key word. Because soon you will not only see yourself "virtually" in your mind, but also for real in the mirror.

And now I wish you much success in achieving your goals!

And don't forget: Always reward yourself for reaching milestones—whatever it may be, treat yourself to something nice, because: You've earned it! But also be "kind" to yourself if things take longer than planned—it's better to add a few more months than to abandon the entire project just because some goals were set too high. Since it's your project, you can of course adjust your goals to your current lifestyle at any time. What's important is that they remain realistic, feasible, and attainable. You decide what you want to see and when. Of course, you can also fill out the tables at times that suit you, more often than after six and twelve months, or at other times that fit your life better—the milestones listed here are just suggestions.

Tip: Take photos of yourself in the mirror, from different but always the same perspectives, to visually document your "journey to becoming slimmer" at the corresponding stages in chronological order. Pictures of your silhouette, your body profile, are wonderful "anchors to long-forgotten times," which can also serve as great "reminders" if you ever lose sight of your goals. A great example of how the "photo album of the melting self" can contribute to success and motivation is the story of 25-year-old insurance broker Alexander, whose diagnosis of obesity prompted him to rethink—and who subsequently lost a whopping 20 kg in 1.5 years by changing his lifestyle. When asked, "How do you feel now when you look in the mirror?" he replied: "When I compare before and after, I'm naturally very proud of myself and know that I'm doing something good for myself and my body. Especially during a motivational slump—which everyone has from time to time—it gives me a boost to look at a before-and-after picture. Friends and family also notice the difference at some point. Of course, you get a lot of positive feedback" (Mertens 2021).

Celebrate your own milestones and always stand by your decisions. And if you think there's a "secret tip"—Alexander says what you hear time and again from those who have successfully lost a lot of weight and kept it off: "There is no secret tip. You have to be motivated yourself to want to change something. Then there are various ways to put it into practice. Everyone has the opportunity—you just have to want it yourself" (Mertens 2021).

Key Points of the Chapter

- Define and document both your milestones and your ultimate goal.
- In addition to "somatic standard parameters" such as weight, waist circumference, etc., also focus on your very own personal goals.
- Take photos of your transformation during your "journey to the new slimmer you."

11.3 Summary: Your Current Level of Knowledge

At this point on your journey to your new desired weight, you now know …

- All diets are based on the same principle: negative energy balance.
- There is no better or worse diet—all diets are the same.
- Most weight loss programs fail and lead to weight gain because they are both impersonal and not tailored to the individual, and are only carried out for a short period.
- The result: the vicious circle/circulus vitiosus:
  (new) diet fails → weight gain → fear of failure/self-doubt → (new) diet fails → …
- Classic diets are therefore considered a "gateway drug" to eating disorders and obesity.
- Trendy diets like low carb and intermittent fasting are no better than other diets, no matter what the media, influencers, and celebrities write and post.
- My new path begins with honest self-awareness: I need to be clear about who I am and what I want. My mindset must align with this. Then I can get started.
- Sustainable weight loss is basically simple at first: With a moderate energy deficit of about 500 kcal per day, you lose about 2 kg per month.
- Find the range of your individual negative energy balance in which you achieve the perfect personal balance between maximum weight loss and minimal sacrifice in the long term.
- How you achieve this negative energy balance is entirely up to you—it depends on your eating preferences and your lifestyle. Essential: The dietary change must suit you, your body, and your daily life; you must feel comfortable with it.
- The "secret key" to staying slim is: keep going and stick with it. Maintain your dietary and lifestyle changes. Your "diet" (which never

really was one) becomes your new lifestyle, which you ideally maintain forever—simply because you feel great with it!

- I DIET MY WAY means: You decide which path you want to take—and you should stick to that path. You can adapt it at any time to your current wishes and needs—or even completely "tailor" it anew if a change in lifestyle requires it. You are the boss in your own ring!
- Create targeted phases and oases of relaxation and self-reflection. Continually update your mindset to the "latest version of yourself."
- Keep moving. It doesn't have to be "real hard-core sports." Choose the activities that you truly enjoy again and again. Freestyle dancing at home is a real option.
- Keep your muscles active with dumbbells.
- And don't forget: The more (new) movements you permanently integrate into your daily life, the better for the long-term, sustainable overall success of the project.
- Do a double SWOT analysis—both of yourself and of your "slimming down" project.
- Check: How close is your project to the ideal version? Also reflect on and document: What else do I expect, what is still personally important to me?
- Keep an "Eat & Feel Diary."
- Document your current eating and drinking habits for 14 days before starting the project.
- **Create a master plan for your goal—including all your milestones and personal visions you want to achieve.**

This concludes the overview. This is now your collected essential knowledge in compact form, which you need for sustainable weight loss. The following chapters will provide you with additional topics to further equip you for your "slimming project" until you reach your goal: your new desired weight.

References

BMEL Bundesministerium für Ernährung und Landwirtschaft: Kompass Ernährung: Einfach leichter essen mit Genuss und ohne Hunger (2019). https://www.in-form.de/fileadmin/Dokumente/Kompass_Ernaehrung/2019-1-kompass-ernaehrung-barrierefrei-neu.pdf. Accessed: 28. Dez. 2020

Mertens K (2021) Alexander (25) hat im Home Gym 20 Kilo abgenommen. https://www.fitbook.de/mind-body/abnehmen-im-lockdown-transformation-alex. Accessed 15. Feb. 2021

12 The Ideal Dietary Change—An Example

If you are still waiting for a specific "diet, recipe, or menu plan" or something similar—there isn't one here. Because this book, due to its individualized approach, does not provide a concrete diet plan to pragmatically work through—simply because there is no "Plan X" that applies to everyone. I DIET MY WAY is the success credo. And no one knows what works best for you personally better than you do.

Regardless, here is a concise overview of the basics of an exemplary, ideal dietary change for weight reduction. This presentation is intended as a "master matrix" for all those who are still looking for some inspiration for their own personal project creation. So then—this is roughly what the path to your desired weight could look like:

Phase 1—Losing Weight to Reach Your New Desired Weight

Daily energy intake
1500 kcal (short-term reduction to 1200 kcal possible)

Calorie deficit/negative energy balance
minus 500 kcal per day (assuming an estimated daily requirement of 2000 kcal)

U. Knop, *Successful and Sustainable Weight Loss*,
https://doi.org/10.1007/978-3-662-72477-4_12

Targeted weight loss//month
2–2.5 kg

Also note:

12.1 Food

Only choose foods that you enjoy eating, that you crave, that taste very good, that your body asks for, that you tolerate well, and that are easy to digest. Do not be afraid of an "unhealthy diet" (see Chaps. 16 and 17).

12.2 Restrictions

None. Everything is allowed within the calorie limit.

12.3 Beverages

Ideally, only calorie-free drinks, as this leaves more energy for (already restricted) food. Note: Fruit juice, soft drinks, alcohol, tea or coffee with milk and sugar—all of these are high-calorie liquids that quickly use up your available calories.

12.4 Meal Times

Always eat when you are most hungry (maximum feel-good feedback from your body). Whether in the morning, at noon, or in the evening, it doesn't matter: eat according to your natural individual chronobiology (i.e., *when* your body develops hunger). The longer the breaks (fasting periods) between meals, the better for your metabolism (autophagy ["cell cleaning"]/physiological basis of intermittent fasting) and the greater your hunger will be. And the greater the hunger, the better the food tastes and the more intense the pleasurable sigh from deep within your belly.

12.5 Culinary Highlight

Treat yourself every day to your personal culinary delight—something extremely delicious that you especially love to eat or drink. Savor this moment of enjoyment just for yourself.

12.6 Meal Frequency

Two main meals of about 600 kcal each and one "culinary highlight per day" (up to 300 kcal)—for example, this could be more than half a bar of chocolate. Important: Celebrate both main meals and the culinary highlight moment with maximum attention and mindfulness, and enjoy them fully with all your senses.

12.7 Specials

On one day of the week, skip a main meal—and in return, really indulge the next day with an extra 600 kcal on your plate. Also "allowed," because basically everything is allowed: Instead of two main meals, just have one meal a day—then really enjoy feeling full and satisfied with up to 1200 kcal at once. This will leave you feeling truly content and full—afterwards, treat yourself to a nice digestive nap like a lion in the savannah. But: that's it for big meals that day.

12.8 Relaxation

Twice a week, do a yoga session or PMR (progressive muscle relaxation) for inner self-reflection on mindset and goals.

12.9 Exercise/Physical Activity

Every day before (and/or after) work, lift weights for 10 minutes (to maintain and build muscle). 10 minutes is enough, don't overdo it. Take a walk during your lunch break. Increase everyday physical activity wherever possible. Plan a bike ride on the weekend. Find an "activity partner" who will join and motivate you!

It can be that simple. If you want it. If you stick with it consistently. Doing—it is and remains the fundamental core verb of the project. Of course, there will be sacrifice and hunger. But not all the time. Long-term hypocaloric dietary changes for weight reduction can, must, and should also offer occasional "oases of indulgent satiety." Carry out Phase 1 for as long as needed and adjust it until you have lost enough weight to reach your desired feel-good weight. Then comes Phase 2.

12.10 Phase 2—Maintaining Your New Desired and Feel-Good Weight

Phase 2 is comparable to Phase 1—except: you can gradually "increase" your daily calories until you feel and see on the scale: "It's too much, I'm gaining weight again." Then reduce your energy intake again. The long-term goal should be that you have gotten to know your body so well that you feel and know at which calorie limit no renewed weight gain occurs (JVG = yo-yo avoidance limit). Until then, you can increase your daily calorie range. Ideally, you will develop a good long-term sense of which foods provide how many calories and when you have reached your "personal limit"—without counting and documenting calories. And: don't forget physical activity. If all this becomes a "flow" that you intuitively enjoy and live out of your own free will and desire, and you don't gain weight again, then the signs are very good that you will maintain your desired weight for a very long time. Maybe even forever. And now: it's your turn! Make of yourself what you wish to become.

12.11 The Five-Step Plan to Achieving Your New Permanent Desired Weight

As a brief chronological guide, the following "Five-Step Plan to Achieving Your New Permanent Desired Weight" can serve as a model path from January to June and "forever"—of course, the start of the six months can be at any time (just as Veganuary or Dry January can also be kicked off in March).

Step I: Honest Self-Reflection/Life Analysis (January)
Who am I, how do I live, how *healthy* am I, why do I look the way I do, why am I/do I feel overweight, which behavioral patterns/routines have led to this; what do I want & why?

Step II: Eating Behavior Analysis (January)
Keep a 14-day journal: What do I eat & drink, when, for what reason, and with what feelings? How much energy do I consume per day?

Step III: Reset Your Mindset! (January/February)
Realignment of personal attitude/thought patterns/mindset and goals: Where do I want to go, which "new me" do I want to see, when, and in what "form"? How do I get there? Which path & what suits me—and what does not?

Step IV: Lifestyle & Dietary Change (February –June)
Develop a new, individually tailored nutrition and lifestyle plan that (forever!) suits me, that I enjoy, and that I look forward to—because it will, with a moderate negative energy balance (about 500 kcal less per day than before) and an expected weight loss of about 2 kg per month, lead to **about 10 kg less body mass** within 5 months by June —and summer can come.

Finally, take a look at the two-part **FAQ video interview on "Focus Online Experts Special"**—here you will once again receive the most important answers to key questions about successful weight loss and maintaining a slim figure, presented in a compact format:

Nutritionist explains the key to achieving your desired weight

Losing weight: Graduate ecotrophologist Uwe Knop reveals the key to success

Key Points of the Chapter

- There is no ideal plan, no perfect blueprint for permanent weight loss that works for everyone.
- If you find it difficult to create your own "becoming lighter" project, then seek inspiration from external sources (such as those mentioned above, and also see Chap. 14).

13

Honest Togetherness vs. Social Media

Two other important questions on your "journey to a new weight" are:

Will I go my way alone, or will I look for a partner or even a "team" with the same goals? And:

Will I share my plans and goals with those around me, with family, friends, or even the public?

13.1 Honestly Together

Regarding the first question: For many people, motivation from like-minded individuals is an enormous booster. You spur each other on to reach the set (milestone) goals and always have a "sparring partner" with whom you can also measure yourself externally (so that your focus is not always solely on yourself). If things are not going as desired, there is someone by your side to build you up and encourage you—and this works both ways, because not only do you receive support, but you also give it, encouraging the other person: that feels good. Ideal partners are therefore good friends or your own partner—because the closer you are, the better the relationship and the emotional connection, the

U. Knop, *Successful and Sustainable Weight Loss*,
https://doi.org/10.1007/978-3-662-72477-4_13

more openly and honestly you can praise, comfort, but also criticize or give a metaphorical kick in the backside. Whether you embark on your "journey to a new slim self" together is a very personal decision. Some prefer to do it alone, others need a partner or even a "weight-loss collective" that assimilates you, so that you lose weight as part of a greater whole—in other words, embedded in a community and not acting "just" for yourself. You should also answer this question for yourself, so that you have reflected on everything and know whether "Lonesome Rider, Dynamic Duo, or Part of the Team" suits you best personally and where you see the greatest long-term and sustainable chances of success for yourself.

13.2 Social Media?

Regarding the second question of "sharing" your journey: You should give this even more thought in advance—especially with regard to social media such as Facebook, X, Instagram & Co. On the one hand, sharing your own transformation has the appeal of showing the public: "Look what I am capable of on my own"—in order to receive gratifying, flattering external validation, to collect likes and words of praise. This is tempting and motivating for many; it can feel like "soothing balm for the soul." However, the flip side of this coin is trolls, haters, and shitstorms. Negative feedback, especially criticism of yourself, personal attacks—these are often harsh "virtual blows to the neck" that not everyone can simply brush off. This often creates enormous external pressure to succeed, and your soul and psyche can suffer greatly as a result—up to and including depressive moods, eating disorders, and self-doubt. Especially in times when things are not going as they should (and those times will come), in these very volatile moments, negative feedback—which often goes below the belt and is malicious and harsh—poses a great danger, not only to the success of your weight loss project itself, but also to your own personality.

Without going into further details or cautionary case studies, let it be said here: Weigh very carefully and wisely whether you want to make your journey to a new slim self public, use social media channels for this, and reveal yourself personally. This double-edged sword can have painful, far-reaching consequences. "The spirits that I called" are then out of the bottle. You should keep that in mind as well.

The Most Important Points of the Chapter

- Be clear about whether you want to lose weight alone, with a partner, or in a team of like-minded people.
- Weigh very carefully whether and to what extent you want to involve others in your "weight loss journey" or let the public participate via social media.

14

Three Who Made It

Before we conclude your "Weight Loss Project," let us present you with three successful "case studies" from 2020 that have clearly demonstrated in public: If you want it, you do it—and you succeed in losing weight. And each person does it in their own individual way, truly in the spirit of I DIET MY WAY. Take the time to look at the stories of Saskia, Günes, and Alexander (either directly via the links in the sources or simply by googling their names and stories)—despite all the differences in their individual lifestyle changes, you will recognize a common denominator of success that unites all three:

> **Want it. Do it. Stick with it. Persevere!**

All three protagonists share a strong will to change their lives. So they take action, become the creators of their new bodies—and persevere, not allowing setbacks to demotivate them, staying the course with their goal always in sight. The insight from the following three "case studies" is as simple as it is plausible and unifying: These individuals

U. Knop, *Successful and Sustainable Weight Loss*,
https://doi.org/10.1007/978-3-662-72477-4_14

independently discovered how it was personally feasible for them to permanently shed unwanted fat. In effect, they developed their own "sustainability diet," tailored it individually to their preferences and lifestyle, and then—did it, that is, successfully implemented it.

Now I wish you interesting insights into the real lives of …

14.1 Success Story 1

Saskia Schilbach (26), intensive care nurse from Heidelberg

In 2017, she was still extremely overweight. She weighed 172 kg. By fall 2020, she had lost almost 100 kg—and not through a "classic" diet or even gastric surgery. Instead, Saskia's MY WAY looked and still looks like this: "I consistently counted calories, treated myself to bread in the evening, pudding in the afternoon, and simply moved more" (Quoos and Geray 2020).

14.2 Success Story 2

Burak Günes (29), paramedic, Mannheim

At age 25, he weighed 200 kg. Today, the scale reads: 90 kg. Burak was so overweight that he was afraid he would no longer be able to save anyone. He decided to change his life. More exercise, better nutrition, a positive attitude—he achieved all this within a year. His credo: "You have to want it" (SWR 2020).

14.3 Success Story 3

Alexander (25), department manager at a health insurance company

After being diagnosed with obesity, Alexander lost 20 kg in just over 1.5 years. There was no "secret": he simply went into a classic calorie deficit and tried to eat better foods. He also set up a small gym at home: two weight benches with a barbell, an EZ curl bar, and two dumbbells—and trained daily. His tip, especially in tough times: "You should just remind yourself what the goal is and not lose sight of it" (Mertens 2021).

Interesting life stories, aren't they? Another thing you hear unanimously from these successful weight-losers: If you haven't experienced it yourself—literally in your own body—it's hard for outsiders to understand how wonderful it feels. It feels as if you are king of the world. And there's something else these people like to report with a beaming smile: "Losing the weight has clearly enabled me to do something that was never possible before: dating and relationships. Since the transformation, I see myself as a fully-fledged, attractive young man who only really catches the eye of many women now" (BILD 2020).

The Most Important Points of the Chapter

- Research success stories on the internet of people who have reached their desired weight by choosing their very own path to their goal—and let yourself be inspired by their I DIET MY WAY stories!
- No matter how different the paths may be, all the "newly slimmed" share the essential trilogy: Want it. Do it. Stick with it. Persevere!

References

BILD (2020) „Diäten haben mich noch dicker gemacht". https://www.bild.de/bild-plus/ratgeber/2020/ratgeber/abnehm-tipps-ohne-diaet-fitnessblogger-deni-verlor-70-kilo-72898820.bild.html. Accessed 16. Feb. 2021

Mertens K (2021) Alexander (25) hat im Home Gym 20 Kilo abgenommen. https://www.fitbook.de/mind-body/abnehmen-im-lockdown-transformation-alex. Accessed on 16.02.2021

Quoos J, Geray A (2020) „Ich habe 100 Kilo abgespeckt". https://www.bild.de/ratgeber/2020/ratgeber/video-doku-saskia-hat-es-satt-ich-habe-100-kilo-abgespeckt-73079360.bild.html. Accessed 16. Feb. 2021

SWR Fernsehen (2020) Burak Günes hat von 200 auf 90 Kilo abgespeckt. https://www.swrfernsehen.de/landesschau-bw/studiogaeste/burak-guenes-hat-von-200-auf-90-kilo-abgespeckt-100.html. Accessed: 16. Feb. 2021

15

Is There a Healthy Diet for Everyone?

The one perfect diet for everyone—it does not exist. What is unhealthy for some may suit others quite well. This applies to every food, to ice cream, and even to white bread. The conclusion: every person deserves their own nutrition plan (Lawton 2020).

This statement opened an article in the journal *Spektrum der Wissenschaft* and it perfectly sums up the current status quo on healthy eating. But why are you reading this here? Quite simply: because it will make it easier for you to choose the foods you can and want to integrate into your new lifestyle. You have complete freedom in shaping your dietary change.

Now that you are well informed about diets and their "universal system of (in)effectiveness and side effects," and perhaps your "get slim project" has already taken shape in your mind, here is a brief digression into the "crystal ball of nutrition research"—because, what few people know: The double credo of nutritional science is: "Nothing is known for certain" and "Nothing but hypotheses." Therefore, the following applies:

U. Knop, *Successful and Sustainable Weight Loss*,
https://doi.org/10.1007/978-3-662-72477-4_15

There is no evidence for *the* healthy diet—just as there is no evidence for healthy or unhealthy foods!

Surprised? Be glad, because this makes it much easier for you to choose the foods you like, that you tolerate well, and that you can fully enjoy with all your senses. Hidden within this is a key element for finding exactly the lifelong diet (or dietary change) that is ideal for you. Because you know: In the long run, only a personal diet that suits you and that you truly enjoy will lead to your desired weight—because only by eating pleasurably and in harmony with your body will you be able to maintain your new eating style permanently.

It is best to forget everything you think you know so far about "healthy eating and unhealthy foods." Because you will be amazed at how outdated this thinking and knowledge from the last millennium seems when you use the current facts as your golden standard for thinking.

15.1 Correlations Are Not Causations

Let's keep it brief: There is no evidence for the widely known and institutionally propagated dietary rules such as "Eating fruits and vegetables five times a day protects against disease," "A high-fiber diet prevents colon cancer," or "Eating little meat is good for the heart," because the foundation of nutrition research is so-called observational studies. And these studies have very weak scientific validity, because:

They cannot provide causality (cause-and-effect relationships), only correlations (statistical associations).

Such associations, in turn, only allow for hypotheses, assumptions, and speculations. A simple example illustrates this system of nutrition research, to which the established system still clings: When it is said,

"Sausage increases the risk of diabetes," only a statistical association between sausage consumption and diabetes risk has been isolated from the study data. Why this association exists, however, no one knows. So no one can say that sausage "increases" the risk of diabetes, but at most: "Sausage eaters have an increased risk." Just as well, one could have found that "carbonated water increases the risk of diabetes," because the data show that people with diabetes drink more sparkling water than still water compared to healthy individuals. That is absurd—and just as absurd are the dietary rules and pyramids of various professional societies, which have been issuing recommendations for a "healthy" diet to the public for decades—and which are not only a popular reference for professionals: Even daycare operators and school principals like to "hide" behind the 10 rules for healthy eating to pressure parents: "Only send your child to school with healthy snacks—we must advise against unhealthy food" (not tolerated in the long run).

Specifically regarding the food pyramids often used as teaching material, the scientist Dr. Jana Meixner, Department of Evidence-Based Medicine and Clinical Epidemiology, Danube University Krems, explained: "Nutrition pyramids attempt to convey a truth about food that does not exist" (Brandstätter 2019).

However, the DGE and professional societies formulate in such "pyramidal" terms because they overinterpret observational studies—for the DGE, these epidemiological investigations are even an "important basis for deriving evidence-based recommendations for the population for the prevention of diet-**re**lated diseases." A side note: Did you notice the little word "related"? Because "diet-caused" alone is too much of a hypothesis even for the nutrition officials, too much of a stretch. But with "related," they gain a lot of interpretive leeway when elevating correlations.

But that aside, because: By elevating observational studies as sources of evidence, the DGE contradicts fundamental research principles, according to which no proof of cause and effect can be derived from nutritional observational studies (epidemiological investigations)—only statistical associations, which always allow only for assumptions. Thus, the scientific consensus is, consequently: Observational studies are not suitable for deriving preventive or therapeutic recommendations.

International criticism of these studies is therefore growing louder, including from within the field of nutritional science itself—but the ever-aging nutrition officials in this country seem to be growing ever more deaf. Even system-critical reviews in professional journals are ignored and remain uncommented. Especially for the hardest of all study endpoints, overall mortality, the evidential value for foods or dietary patterns is zero. Nor is there even a hint of evidence for the effect of diet in preventing disease. To summarize again:

There is neither causal evidence for reducing mortality nor for the primary prevention of diseases through diet.

Research in this area appears hopeless. More and more publications of this "persuasion" support the critical statements of numerous international scientists.

Even the German *Ärzte-Zeitung* warned in early 2014 to exercise greater caution when interpreting nutritional observational studies. An editorial denounced "many studies with little substance": "There is an abundance of studies on how to eat healthily. But most should be treated with the utmost caution. With observational studies, it can only be determined whether two situations occur together more frequently. But from such a coincidence, no causal relationship can be derived." It continues: "Only with huge long-term studies under randomized controlled conditions will it ultimately be possible to find out which diet can reduce mortality. Such studies are extremely complex and expensive" (Schumacher 2014). And not only that: Such nutrition studies are practically impossible to conduct, which is why there are no relevant high-quality studies, so-called RCTs (Randomized Clinical Trials) with long durations (5–10 years or more), that can causally demonstrate hard clinical endpoints with dose-response relationships and can be reproduced in other comparable RCTs. As a side note: Reproducibility of RCTs is the "core currency" of scientific knowledge. These gold standard studies, which provide robust causalities, are conducted in nutrition research, but:

Nutrition RCTs are extremely limited in their validity, as they are too short, include too few participants, usually do not reveal a clear dose-response relationship, and are not confirmed in further RCTs. In short: Valid long-term data on hard endpoints such as stroke, heart attack, and death are lacking.

Especially with the "big nutritional questions" of humanity, there is a major problem: If one wanted to research whether, for example, a vegetarian diet is healthier than a diet including meat, the effort would fail right at the start—because even the most important study criterion, "randomization," cannot be implemented. Yet this random allocation of participants to different study groups is essential to ensure balance and comparability of the groups, to exclude confounding factors that could distort results, and to obtain scientifically robust findings. However, no one is willing to be told for two, five, or even ten years of study duration that they must not eat meat because they were assigned to the vegetarian group—conversely, one can hardly imagine the outcry if vegetarians were assigned to the meat group for ten years …

In this context, the so-called "flagship RCT" named PREDIMED should be mentioned, which nutrition advocates finally cite as "real evidence" for the health benefits of the Mediterranean diet, said to offer optimal protection against cardiovascular disease. Unfortunately, this extremely weak RCT does not allow for such far-reaching conclusions by any means. Due to numerous weaknesses, limitations, and inconsistencies, the "great results" of PREDIMED were at the time named the "Unstatistic of the Month" by the RWI (Leibniz Institute for Economic Research, Essen) (Gigerenzer 2014)—that is, exposed as untenable, because the study's results were misrepresented or exaggerated in public communications (in PR, in the media). Furthermore, the PREDIMED study was retracted due to problems, especially with the crucial randomization, and then republished (Kron 2019), which further weakens its already limited validity.

For the sake of completeness, it should be mentioned: There was—hard to believe—13 years ago a truly serious 8-year long-term RCT with almost 50,000 US women (aged 50–79), who were randomized into two groups ("healthy diet" [including lots of fruits and vegetables] and a comparison group without "dietary intervention") and examined for numerous cardiovascular disease parameters. In 2006, this study was published in one of the top three scientific journals, *JAMA* (Howard et al. 2006). Prof. Ingrid Mühlhauser, health scientist at the University of Hamburg and chair of the German Network for Evidence-Based Medicine, stated clearly: "The only really good study, with a large number of participants and over eight years, found that it made absolutely no difference how the subjects ate. Cancer, heart attack, stroke, diabetes—all the same" (Treuer and Suckow 2020). Since then, no comparably good nutrition study has been published … but thousands more epidemiological investigations have appeared.

15.2 Criticism of Observational Studies Remains Unabated

As early as mid-2017, the *Ärzte-Zeitung* once again made it clear in light of this flood of observational studies: "A causal relationship cannot be proven by nutritional studies. The influence of numerous factors [confounders = 'lifestyle confounding factors'] can only be incompletely eliminated in observational studies." In another article, the question was raised as to whether nutritional observational studies amount to "epidemiological fortune-telling with coffee grounds" (Borchers 2017). In the same year, a major German pharmacy magazine titled a critical article on the universally popular misinterpretation of observational research "Tempting Nonsense"—simply because it is all too easy to calculate the highly complex interconnections, statistically sound mind you, and then sell this nonsense as truth. This confusion of cause and effect, and thus the erroneous inference of causality, is a chronic, ineradicable error in the evaluation of such studies.

The universal credo of nutritional science is therefore, quite logically—you already know it: We know nothing for sure!

15.3 If You Don't Eat, You Die

No question, of course there are causal relationships between health and disease and nutrition… It would be presumptuous and biologically-physiologically unwise to deny this, because eating and nutrition are far too fundamental. Food keeps body and soul together. Eating "our daily bread" several times is in fact the most basic (instinctive) behavior for survival. Without food, we die—clear causal evidence! But: The causal relationships with "healthy nutrition (philosophy)" so fervently desired by ideologically motivated hardliners cannot be evaluated, measured, or (causally) established—simply because the entire system of nutrition is too individual and highly complex, and the necessary studies are simply not feasible—neither today nor tomorrow. And this is unacceptable both for the self-image of the nutritional science system and for the "believers in the many better-eating hypes." Ergo, things are exaggerated, fantasized, and wishful thinking is stylized as truth—so that the mantra becomes: "We know what's going on and we'll tell you what you should and shouldn't do. So listen to us if you care about your health!"

But the crucial question must be: If you don't like something, if you don't tolerate it well, if it upsets your stomach, it can't be healthy—what does your common sense say? Ergo, there can be no "healthy diet for everyone," because every person has different preferences and aversions, determined by genes, individual metabolism, and phase-dependent lifestyle. One person likes fish, another almost vomits at the smell. One tolerates a lot of raw food and indigestible fiber, another gets nasty flatulence, a bloated belly, cramps, and pain from it…

The fact that this opinion is not an "exotic exclusive view" of the author of this book is made clear and unambiguous by the steadily growing, concerted opinion of numerous international scientists—both in scientific publications and in media statements. Because: Nutritional research is like reading a crystal ball. It sounds harsh, but that's how it must be seen objectively and free of ideology. Just as, for example, Prof. Dirk Haller sees it, Chair of Nutrition and Immunology at the Weihenstephan Science Center (WZW) and Director of ZIEL,

Institute for Food & Health, an interdisciplinary central institute at the Technical University of Munich:

"At the moment, there is a huge era of correlations in this field—and the fact that it is correlative means that you can actually say very little. Therefore, the order of the day is to give no specific advice at all regarding healthy nutrition." (Spektrum 2017)

Interestingly, as early as a year before, Prof. Peter Stehle, former board member of the DGE e. V. (German Nutrition Society), had clearly stated:

"We cannot provide sufficient scientific evidence. The observed results of nutritional research are therefore, of course, very, very weak in terms of argumentation. But that has always been the case and will remain so. The influence of nutrition on health (condition) cannot be quantified. Nobody knows." (Rosenkranz 2016)

Nutritional physician Prof. Hans Konrad Biesalski, University of Hohenheim, puts it succinctly: "In fact, even today, no one knows what really constitutes a healthy meal for the average person" (Friebe 2017).

Thus, the consistent demand of Prof. John P. Ioannidis—medical statistician, Stanford University, one of the most cited scientists of all time—is entirely understandable: "Nutritional studies are full of methodological flaws and therefore not meaningful. Ergo, I recommend to the authors of nutritional studies: Start all over again!" (Lutterotti 2018).

Let us return to the opening quote of the chapter and close the circle of ignorance with another statement from the first-cited article: "To this day, nutritional science cannot provide a concrete answer to perhaps the most pressing question: What constitutes a healthy diet?" (Lawton 2020).

Quite simply: There are as many healthy diets as there are people, because: Everyone is different.

Key Points of the Chapter

- There is no evidence for a "healthy" diet for everyone, because research must rely on scientifically highly limited observational studies.
- However, these epidemiological investigations, by their very nature, do not provide evidence (causal evidence), but only vague associations (correlations) that allow only hypotheses and assumptions.

- That is why this field of research is, quite rightly, subject to massive criticism and a call for (its) radical reform.
- So free yourself from the compulsion to live up to a "healthy" diet. Instead, the following applies:
- There are as many healthy diets as there are people, because: Everyone is different.

References

Borchers M (2017) Ernährungsstudien—Epidemiologische Kaffeesatzleserei? https://www.aerztezeitung.de/Medizin/Epidemiologische-Kaffeesatzleserei-303951.html. Accessed 4. Sept. 2020

Brandstätter G (2019) Der Mythos von der gesunden Ernährung. https://www.derstandard.de/story/2000100630455/der-mythos-von-der-gesunden-ernaehrung. Accessed 4. Sept. 2020

Friebe R (2017) Eine einzige fette Lüge. https://www.faz.net/aktuell/wissen/medizin-ernaehrung/low-fat-diaet-eine-einzige-fette-luege-15202206.html. Accessed 4. Sept. 2020

Gigerenzer G (2014) Olivenöl verhindert Diabetes. https://www.rwi-essen.de/unstatistik/27/. Accessed 4. Sept. 2020

Howard et al (2006) Low-fat dietary pattern and risk of cardiovascular disease: the Women's Health Initiative Randomized Controlled Dietary Modification Trial. JAMA 295(6):655–666. https://doi.org/10.1001/jama.295.6.655

Kron T (2019) Ernährung bei Diabetes—Was gesichert ist und was nicht. https://www.diqm.de/article/195966. Accessed 4. Sept. 2020

Lawton G (2020) Die eine perfekte Ernährung für alle gibt es nicht. https://www.spektrum.de/news/ernaehrung-das-gesunde-essen-fuer-uns-alle-gibt-es-nicht/1799795. Accessed on 24.12.2020

Lutterotti N (2018) Ins Essen verbissen—was eine gesunde Ernährung ist, darüber lässt sich genüsslich streiten. https://www.nzz.ch/wissenschaft/ins-essen-verbissen-was-eine-gesunde-ernaehrung-ist-darueber-laesst-sich-genuesslich-streiten-ld.1410288. Accessed 4. Sept. 2020

Rosenkranz M (2016) Der Verbraucher versteht das Wort Risiko nicht. https://ga.de/ratgeber/fit-und-gesund/der-verbraucher-versteht-das-wort-risiko-nicht_aid-42678869. Accessed 4. Sept. 2020

Schumacher B (2014) Leitartikel zur Ernährung—Viele Studien mit wenig Nährwert. https://www.aerztezeitung.de/Medizin/Viele-Studien-mit-wenig-Naehrwert-238585.html. Accessed 4. Sept. 2020

Spektrum (2017) Das Abnehm-Paradox. https://www.spektrum.de/video/das-abnehm-paradox/1512991. Accessed 4. Sept. 2020

Treuer M. Suckow M (2020) Gesunde Ernährung—Was dürfen wir alles essen? https://www1.wdr.de/fernsehen/die-story/sendungen/gesunde-ernaehrung-134.html. Accessed 4. Sept. 2020

Further Reading

Lesenswerte Literaturhinweise: Wer sich noch intensiver in die zahlreichen Schwächen und in die immer lauter werdende Kritik an der Ernährungsforschung einarbeiten möchte, dem seien folgende Publikationen ans „Ernährungsherz" gelegt

Penders et al (2017) Capable and credible? Challenging nutrition science. Eur J Nutr 56(6):2009–2012. https://doi.org/10.1007/s00394-017-1507-y. (Ein wunderbares niederländisches Plädoyer für die „Neuerfindung der Ernährungswissenschaft")

Ioannidis J (2018) The challenge of reforming nutritional epidemiologic research. JAMA 320(10):969–970. https://doi.org/10.1001/jama.2018.11025. (Zwar nur zwei Seiten umfassend, aber die haben es in sich: Es geht um nicht weniger als die „Radikalreform der Ernährungsforschung")

Maki et al (2014) Limitations of observational evidence: implications for evidence-based dietary recommendations. Adv Nutr 5(1):7–15. https://doi.org/10.3945/an.113.004929. (Politiker, seid vorsichtig mit Ernährungsempfehlungen, denn es fehlt die Evidenz)

Wlison C (2019) Was sollen wir essen? https://www.spektrum.de/kolumne/was-sollen-wir-essen/1685738. (Ein höchst informativer Rundumschlag, der den Finger richtig tief in die Wunde der Limitierungen und Schwächen der Ernährungsforschung legt)

16

The Classification Into Healthy and Unhealthy Foods Is ...

Now that you know that evidence for healthy nutrition—in the sense of causal evidence—does not exist, you may still be asking yourself the following question: What about healthy and unhealthy foods? At least here, can a clear distinction be made? Generally, it is said: fast food, sweets, white bread, and fatty meats—these are the unhealthy foods. Whole grain bread, fish, and of course plenty of fruits and vegetables, these categories belong in the "healthy" basket. But, as you may already suspect…

So, if you are among those who have so far happily or dutifully oriented yourself by the clear "division into healthy and unhealthy foods"—then you should brace yourself, because the following statements may shake your worldview a little.

So now read the current statements from the five leading international "D-A-CH state nutrition authorities" (Knop 2019):

Quote

"We do not need rigid rules or a division into healthy or unhealthy foods. What matters is how much of what I eat."

U. Knop, *Successful and Sustainable Weight Loss*,
https://doi.org/10.1007/978-3-662-72477-4_16

Harald Seitz, Head of Public Relations, Federal Center for Nutrition (BZfE) (March 2019)

Quote

"We find the general division into healthy and unhealthy difficult. Whether a food is ultimately healthy or unhealthy is determined by the amount consumed."

Sonja Schäche, Head of Press and Public Relations, German Institute of Human Nutrition Potsdam-Rehbrücke (DIfE) (March 2019)

Quote

"There are no forbidden foods. The combination of foods in the right proportions makes for a balanced diet."

Thomas Krienbühl, Communications Specialist, Swiss Society for Nutrition SGE (March 2019)

Quote

"Foods should not be classified as 'healthy' or 'unhealthy.' What matters for a balanced diet are the quantity, combination, and preparation of foods."

Mag. Alexandra Hofer, Managing Director, Austrian Nutrition Society (ÖGE) (March 2019)

Quote

"We do not consider a division into healthy and unhealthy foods to be meaningful. What matters is how much of what I eat."

Antje Gahl, Head of Public Relations, German Nutrition Society (DGE) (March 2019)

And that's not all—even the two major associations of ecotrophologists from Germany and Austria share the same opinion:

"To speak of 'healthy' or 'unhealthy' foods falls short given the complexity of nutrition. Populist recommendations of individual so-called 'healthy' foods or even bans on supposedly 'unhealthy' foods are rather counterproductive and can lead to consumer confusion." (Dr. Andrea Lambeck, Managing Director, Professional Association of Ecotrophologists (VDOE)) (May 2019)

"The relationship between people and food is too complex to derive a helpful classification into good and bad foods." (Mag. Andreas Schmölzer, First Chairman, Association of Nutrition Scientists Austria (VEÖ)) (May 2019)

And so the consensus is: A division into healthy and unhealthy foods is not possible, as scientific evidence is lacking.

With these statements, everything on this topic should be said—or so one might think. Unfortunately, these two outdated categories of "healthy and unhealthy" are still used for foods. The question is: Do the authors neither know about the lack of evidence nor about the crystal-clear statements from the professional organizations? Or do they simply not want to accept it, in line with the health apostles' motto: What must not be, cannot be…

Now you know better. And to further deepen your understanding, here are some highly recommended recent publications from 2020, whose findings fit perfectly into the picture and unequivocally reinforce previous research and statements. But first, a fitting statement from one of Germany's most renowned nutrition scientists:

"The influence of individual foods is so small that, compared to other factors, it simply does not matter." (Hannelore Daniel, nutritional physiologist and emeritus professor at the Technical University of Munich; Russo 2020)

16.1 Identical Meals—Different Reactions

Just as there are no healthy foods for everyone, because the important 3Ds (digestion, utilization, and tolerance) are always individually different, people also do not all react the same way to the same food. Here, too, it is repeatedly shown: The body's reactions are completely different. A comprehensive publication on this appeared as early as June 2020 in the renowned journal *Nature Medicine* (Berry et al. 2020). Scientists at King's College London studied more than 1,100 adults from the UK and the USA, including several hundred pairs of twins. The target parameters measured and documented were the release of the "sugar hormone" insulin and the rise in blood sugar and fat levels in response to precisely defined, identical meals for all participants.

The results showed: Individuals' metabolic responses to the same meal are often very different. The researchers found that there are large individual differences among participants in their physical metabolic responses after eating. "Blood fats, blood sugar (glucose), and the hormone insulin vary after identical meals." The London researchers concluded: "It is increasingly clear that general dietary recommendations are not suitable for everyone" (Lawton 2020). This study is the most comprehensive assessment to date of metabolic responses to identical meals in a rigorous, well-controlled study design. Furthermore, due to the significant inter-individual differences observed in metabolic responses to the same meals, standardized dietary recommendations that apply to everyone must be completely questioned. For the authors, their results mean that personalized nutrition could have real potential for disease prevention. One of the authors, Prof. Tim Spector, also made it clear: "We have moved away from the idea that there is a healthy standard diet for everyone."

16.2 Paradigm Shift in Nutrition Research

The conclusion of the *Pharmazeutische Zeitung* (Rösler 2020), which reported on the study, is accordingly clear: "Whether sugar, fat, or other nutrients: According to a new study, the way the body reacts to different foods varies so much from person to person that general dietary recommendations seem pointless … The first lesson to be drawn from these results is: There is no one diet that is ideal for everyone." That's exactly how it is. Consequently, shortly thereafter, another publication in the top journal *JAMA* made it clear: "The modern view of food and medicine has led to a significant shift in nutrition research and practice, toward precision nutrition" (Rogers and Collins 2020). Precision nutrition refers to the tailored nutrition of the individual. For the *JAMA* authors, this new form of "precise nutrition" is the answer to: what one must eat to stay healthy. According to Germany's most renowned fasting medicine expert, Prof. Andreas Michalsen of Charité Berlin, this could also be the future of nutritional counseling: "Perhaps in the end we will stick to personalized diets and no longer give any general recommendations" (Borgeest and Boytchev 2021).

Therefore, you can be sure: The paradigm shift in nutritional science has begun—and it is irreversible; on the contrary, it is advancing rapidly. General, off-the-shelf rules have melted away to small puddles of "yesterday's snow." Individualized nutrition is and will be the eating trend of the future. The top U.S. health authorities, the National Institutes of Health, have also defined the core topic of personalized nutrition ("precision nutrition") as a central focus of their new strategic research plan for 2020–2030 (NHI 2020). The topic is also gaining momentum in Germany: As part of the funding for competence clusters in nutrition research, four junior research groups are being supported by the Federal Ministry of Education and Research to scientifically analyze personalized nutrition from different perspectives (Holzapfel et al. 2021).

16.3 Everyone Is (and Eats) Different

As new and surprising as the aforementioned findings may sound—the fact that individuals have different metabolic responses to comparable meals has long been known and described. The new *Nature* paper confirms the findings of an extensive Israeli study from the Weizmann Institute of Science, which was already published in the journal *Cell* in 2015 (Zeevi et al. 2015):

Through elaborate experiments conducted under standardized and well-controlled conditions, the researchers discovered that different people react very differently to the same food. In the study, blood and stool samples were analyzed, and the development of blood sugar levels in over 800 participants was measured after eating. The rise in blood sugar showed, regardless of the meal, independent and sometimes completely individual patterns—even after a standardized breakfast, for example. Or there was the following phenomenon: In some participants, blood sugar rose more after eating sushi than after eating ice cream, while in other study participants, the exact opposite reaction was documented. However, in individual participants, no different reaction to the same food was observed on different days. The study used mobile blood glucose monitors and smartphone apps to consistently and seamlessly document measurements and eating behavior. Ultimately, blood sugar responses to almost 50,000 meals could be evaluated. The conclusion: The human body processes the same foods in very different, individual ways. But the sheer extent of these differences surprised even the researchers: "That was a huge surprise. We never expected differences of this magnitude," recalls Prof. Christian Sina, head of the Institute of Nutritional Medicine at the University Hospital of Lübeck (Herden 2020).

This fits with the insight from previous chapters: There are as many healthy diets as there are people, because everyone is (and eats) different. The Israeli study leader, Prof. Eran Elinav of the Weizmann Institute of Science in Israel, stated: "At the same time, we learned something very interesting but also unsettling: that the paradigm of healthy eating is fundamentally wrong" (Lawton 2020).

Let us finally allow Germany's "number one official nutrition authority," the German Nutrition Society (DGE), to clarify that eating does not have to be made into a science. DGE spokesperson Antje Gahl emphasized this during coverage of nutrition in the time of coronavirus (dpa/FAZ 2020). Even the Scientific Advisory Board for Agricultural Policy, Nutrition, and Consumer Health Protection at the Federal Ministry of Food and Agriculture stated clearly and unequivocally in its 2020 report on "Policy for More Sustainable Nutrition": "The evidence that certain foods or food groups have a positive or negative effect on certain non-communicable diseases is low" (WBAE 2020).

In this spirit: Create and enjoy your very own healthy diet—one that tastes delicious to you for the rest of your life, does you good, and keeps you sustainably slim.

Personalized dietary recommendations are now also being intensively discussed in the nutritional science literature on weight reduction. "The *one size fits all* approach to weight loss has been increasingly criticized in recent years, both in society and among experts, and is no longer up to date. Tailored dietary recommendations are on the rise" (Holzapfel et al. 2021). The authors of this German publication further state clearly that the literature shows people react very differently to foods and that, by definition, there cannot be a single dietary recommendation for weight loss. That's exactly how it is. I DIET MY WAY is the only successful path to the goal. The researchers at TU Munich also offer a very important piece of advice: Save your money on genetic tests, blood, proteome, and microbiome analyses that claim to make weight loss easier! Because:

"Currently, it is not possible to provide personalized, evidence-based dietary recommendations based on a person's genetic makeup or the composition of their gut microbiota." (Holzapfel et al. 2021)

The reason, as always, is quick and easy to explain: To this day (2025), there is no scientific evidence (causal evidence) for a clinically relevant connection between genetic factors or the gut microbiota (formerly "gut flora") and the intensity or success of weight loss. The same applies to various blood tests and metabolic analyses that examine the so-called proteome (protein compounds in the cells): Here, too, no evidence-based transfer for personal dietary recommendations can be derived—neither for healthy eating nor for weight loss.

Ergo: Don't fall for the scientifically baseless promises of commercial providers. Instead, spend your money on high-quality foods of the best quality that you truly enjoy eating. The lack of evidence for all kinds of tests for personalized nutrition makes it even clearer what really matters:

What is absolutely crucial is complete trust in your own body. Because only your body knows the personalized diet that is best and healthiest for you—no one else does.

Key Points of the Chapter

- It is not possible to categorize foods as healthy or unhealthy, as scientific evidence is lacking.
- Personalized, individual nutrition is the trend of the future ("Precision Nutrition").
- Avoid commercial genetic, proteome, and microbiome analyses for weight loss and/or personalized nutrition—there is no scientific evidence for their "assistance."
- Therefore, with a clear "scientific" conscience, choose only the foods for your dietary change that you truly like—this is one of the key success factors for sticking with it in the long term.

References

Berry et al (2020) Human postprandial responses to food and potential for precision nutrition. Nat Med 26:964–973. https://doi.org/10.1038/s41591-020-0934-0

Borgeest M, Boytchev H (2021) Ernährung als Glaubensfrage. https://www.focus.de/gesundheit/ernaehrung/spezialisten-im-streitgespraech-ernaehrung-als-glaubensfrage_id_12871498.html. Accessed 15. Feb. 2021

dpa/FAZ (2020) Deutsche legen in Pandemie an Gewicht zu. https://www.faz.net/aktuell/gesellschaft/gesundheit/coronavirus/deutsche-legen-in-pandemie-kraeftig-an-gewicht-zu-17006072.html. Accessed 17. Oct. 2020

Herden B (2020) Das Ende der Diätregeln, wie wir sie kennen. https://www.welt.de/wissenschaft/plus219635612/Stoffwechsel-Das-Ende-der-Diaetregeln-wie-wir-sie-kennen.html. Accessed 25. Dec. 2020

Holzapfel et al (2021) Personalized dietary recommendations for weight loss. A scientific perspective from various angles. Ernaehrungs Umschau 68(2):26–35. https://doi.org/10.4455/eu.2021.008

Knop U (2019) Dein Körpernavigator zum besten Essen aller Zeiten. Polarise-Verlag, Heidelberg

Lawton G (2020) Die eine perfekte Ernährung für alle gibt es nicht. https://www.spektrum.de/news/ernaehrung-das-gesunde-essen-fuer-uns-alle-gibt-es-nicht/1799795. Accessed 24. Dec. 2020

NHI (2020) National Institutes of Health: 2020–2030 strategic plan for NIH nutrition research. A report of the NIH nutrition research task force. http://www.niddk.nih.gov/about-niddk/strategic-plans-reports/strategic-plan-nih-nutrition-research. Accessed 24. Dec. 2020

Rogers G, Collins F (2020) Precision nutrition – the answer to „what to eat to stay healthy". JAMA 324(8):735–736. https://doi.org/10.1001/jama.2020.13601

Rösler A (2020) Diäten – Eine für alle gibt es nicht. https://www.pharmazeutische-zeitung.de/eine-fuer-alle-gibt-es-nicht-118970/. Accessed 4. Sept. 2020

Russo S (2020) Ernährungsforschung – Woran Ernährungsstudien scheitern. https://www.higgs.ch/woran-ernaehrungsstudien-scheitern/38733/. Accessed 31. Dec. 2020

WBAE (2020) Politik für eine nachhaltigere Ernährung: Eine integrierte Ernährungspolitik entwickeln und faire Ernährungsumgebungen gestalten – WBAE-Gutachten. https://www.bmel.de/SharedDocs/Downloads/DE/_Ministerium/Beiraete/agrarpolitik/wbae-gutachten-nachhaltige-ernaehrung.pdf;jsessionid=FD60238BE2E6A9BCF3C6B52A24344AE8.internet2842?__blob=publicationFile&v=3. Accessed 25. Dec. 2020

Zeevi et al (2015) Personalized nutrition by prediction of glycemic responses. Cell 163(5):1079–1094. https://doi.org/10.1016/j.cell.2015.11.001

17 The Natural Diet Alternative: Intuitive Eating

Now we have reached the point where you know everything you need to know to make your decision: Do I begin my lifelong lifestyle modification for targeted weight loss, that is, do I make a long-term change to my diet (and other areas of my life), and if so, how—or not? You now know not only about the "crystal ball" approach to nutrition and the lack of evidence for both healthy eating in general and for healthy and unhealthy foods. Most importantly, you are now informed about the core topic of this book and your reason for reading it: How do all diets work, what really matters, what is fake, what is fact, where are the opportunities, where are the risks—and where do I stand in this "decision matrix"? You have been transparently and scientifically objectively informed, so you can now form your own opinion—to answer the crucial weight-related question for yourself, openly and honestly: Do I want to lose weight in a targeted way and stay slim(mer) in the long term, in other words, is my credo I DIET MY WAY? Am I fully aware of the path I am choosing? If your answer is "Yes, I do!", then you can actually skip the following chapter—unless you are curious about the most natural form of human nutrition: intuitive eating.

U. Knop, *Successful and Sustainable Weight Loss*,
https://doi.org/10.1007/978-3-662-72477-4_17

For all other readers who are still uncertain after reading, or who are already clear and at peace with themselves that they would rather not get on the "weight loss carousel," the following presents an alternative path: **Eat intuitively and achieve your biological feel-good weight!**

Let's start at the beginning: What does it actually mean to "eat intuitively"? At its core, it's quite simple: On the one hand, you eat with complete (self-)trust, relying only on your own body.

> Hunger, desire, satiety, and tolerance are the new guiding emotions that lead you to the enjoyable, life-sustaining food your body loves—because it needs it.

On the other hand, you no longer listen to advice or advisors telling you what is good or bad for you. At first, this may sound rather "incredibly exotic"—to simply stop following any rules about healthy eating. But intuitive eating (IE) is by no means an insider tip anymore—even the government has now recognized that we are talking here about the most original and natural form of human nutrition.

For example, the Baden-Württemberg State Center for Nutrition describes IE as follows: "Just listen to your gut feeling! Imagine if there were no more rules, regulations, or restrictions when it comes to eating. Just indulge and enjoy whatever you feel like… an unreasonable dream? No, a model with health and success potential!" Intuitive eating, a relatively young theory, is described as a counter-concept to modern eating philosophies (full of imposed restrictions)—in other words, as an "anti-diet." Intuitive eating is not a revolutionary idea, but rather a return to the essentials, to the most natural way of eating, which many people have lost over the course of their lives. "It's about not constantly worrying about your meal plan" (Lück 2019).

If we look one level higher from the "Ländle" to the Federal Center for Nutrition (BZfE), which is part of the Federal Office for Agriculture and Food (BLE) and supports the Federal Ministry of Food and Agriculture, we learn the following about IE:

> "No more diets, no nutrition rules, no distinction between healthy or unhealthy, allowed or forbidden: with so-called intuitive eating, our body is supposed to tell us what is good for us." (Freitag-Ziegler 2019)

But that is often easier said than done, because for that, we also have to listen to our body—and correctly understand its signals. Some people have lost this ability today. They no longer eat with trust in their gut feeling, but out of habit, sociability, frustration, or boredom. Or—perhaps you recognize yourself—they ignore their growling stomach because they want to lose weight.

Anyone who no longer knows their body must reestablish the connection to their innermost self. Because only those who can hear and listen to their body, who can correctly interpret the emotions and inner signals, will find that IE becomes a true source of self-love—for only by eating in harmony with body and mind, with soul and emotions, do we achieve the highest level of integrity with ourselves—as well as our biological, natural feel-good weight.

17.1 Eat Mindfully What Does You Good!

Because no food and no meal that we do not enjoy can be healthy and good for our weight—otherwise, our body would not consistently reject it right at the first checkpoint called the mouth. Food that our organism "does not approve of taste-wise" is not good for it. And that is exactly what it should be, because "doing good" is slowly but surely becoming the official basic consensus. "We should learn to trust our basic feeling again, listen more to our own body, and learn to reflect on what tastes good to us and what really does us good. We don't need rigid rules or a classification into healthy or unhealthy foods for that. What matters is how much of what I eat. Of course, enjoyment should not be neglected," recommends nutritionist Dr. Margareta Büning-Fesel, who heads the Federal Center for Nutrition (BZfE) (Müller 2019).

The new "national health portal" of the federal government (https://gesund.bund.de), where citizens have been able to find information about common diseases and numerous preventive measures since September 2020, also makes it clear in its mandatory tips for healthy eating (gesund.bund 2020):

> "Important to know: In addition, when it comes to nutrition, you should always listen to your own body. Questions like: What does me good, what do I tolerate better or worse, after which food do I feel sluggish or energized? can help."

This advice, too, is a clear, albeit indirect, state-certified recommendation for more intuition in eating. And with that, you also maximize the likelihood that your body will settle permanently and consistently at its biological desired weight, its natural feel-good weight. And that is exactly the counter-concept to diets—though sometimes it still helps with weight loss...

17.2 IE = Desired & Feel-Good Weight?

> In 2019, Swiss scientists showed in the world's first meta-analysis of IE studies that with intuitive eating confidence and mindful nutrition, you can lose weight just as well as with classic diets.

For their publication in *Obesity Reviews*, the Zurich researchers analyzed only controlled studies (10) on eating patterns based on mindful and intuitive nutrition, and compared them both with non-diet populations and with people who had been on a diet (Artiles et al. 2019). They found two things: First, a significant weight loss with mindful and intuitive eating strategies compared to the control group that did not diet. Furthermore, the authors compared IE with "classic diet forms": With both nutritional approaches, participants lost about the same amount of weight. At first, this all sounds quite nice, but the absolute weight loss figures are rather moderate—on average, about 350 g. The difference between the IE population and the non-diet population was therefore not very large. Nevertheless, it is statistically significant. Because: One must distinguish between the individual level and the population level. As an individual, a weight loss of 348 g is not very much. But if an entire population moves by that much on average, it means that some do not lose any weight, others lose much more. So it is nothing more and nothing less than the average value of all. The difference between the IE population and the diet population was actually 0.0, that is, nothing. This means that, on average, both populations lost exactly the same amount of weight—both about these few hundred grams on average. Again, this means: Some lost nothing, others lost a lot.

Even though the results of the meta-analysis showed that intuitive eating reduces weight comparably to conventional diets, and the authors conclude in their paper that IE could be a "practical approach to weight control," one should not have false hopes when starting IE. Because IE is not a diet, it does not automatically lead to (significant) weight loss. That is something everyone should know. It is possible to lose weight, some may lose a lot, others little or nothing—just as in the Swiss study. A slight weight gain is also possible—depending on how restrictive your previous eating habits were.

17.3 Viva la Feel-Good Weight!

However, it is most likely that healthy individuals will reach their biological feel-good weight—but this happens entirely free from diet stress, instead full of freedom in eating.

> Only those who choose the right path for themselves to their personal feel-good weight will feel truly comfortable in the long term. And that is more important than the number on the scale.

And everyone can only find this out for themselves—in their own personal IE self-experiment. If you have chosen IE as your basic preferred eating style, you can expect the following:

This evolutionarily most natural way of eating can lead not only to a feel-good weight, but also to greater quality of life, joy, pleasure, and satisfaction, as well as increased feelings of self-worth and self-love. And that is what ultimately matters. However, you should let go of the pure desire to lose weight through IE—because that can raise hopes that may remain unfulfilled at the end of the day. Even though the Swiss study was not the first to observe success in weight reduction through IE.

17.4 A Saint Bernard will Never be a Greyhound

The basic rule is: About 70–80% of our body weight is estimated to be genetically determined. Nature always wants diversity within a species, and so we are born thick or thin and in all weight classes in between. So if you are healthy, listen to your body when eating, and do not fit the current model template visually, it is likely due to your genetic makeup. If you want to reduce this, your natural weight, you should know: You are starting a battle against your own body, which can only be won in the long term with the right mindset, strength, stamina, and perseverance. Classic diets should definitely be avoided, as between 80 and 90% of all weight loss attempts fail. Many people even end up heavier afterwards. You already know all this.

17.5 Where There's a will, is There a Way?

But a few manage to do what many dream of in vain forever: They plan to lose weight, follow through with the project, and lose weight—and: They then remain permanently at this new level. One thing is clear: Anyone can lose weight, but maintaining the reduced weight is the real challenge. For all those who have tried countless diets unsuccessfully and have only gotten heavier instead of thinner, the question naturally arises: What do the successful weight-losers do differently? What flipped their "magical mindset switch"? What life-changing experience made it click? Why does someone reinvent themselves, literally shed their old self, and create a new identity? Only the "successfully affected" can answer these questions, because here an individual mix of biology (genes/metabolism/set point), environment, social factors, psychology (willpower/resilience), and energetics (calorie balance) plays the decisive role. One thing is certain for all successful individuals: They have committed to a lifelong "ego relaunch project." Their will to fundamentally change their lives was the top priority, and the decision to invest a lot of energy and time in the "new slim self" was unshakeable. Whether this path will ultimately be sustainable and, above all, lead to greater satisfaction and health remains to be seen.

17.6 Eliminate Emotional Eating!

Whatever personal reasons were decisive for lasting fat loss success, these always individual success stories can only be copied in a rudimentary way, because there is no universal recipe for the noble goal of "staying slim permanently, maintaining reduced weight in the long term." However, anyone who wants to lose weight should have an answer to the question: Why am I actually eating right now? Because:

A central role in weight development and reduction is played by eating without hunger, that is, emotional eating.

Therefore, before starting a diet or changing your eating habits, you should first examine your life for situations in which you eat "compensatorily"—that is, not out of real hunger, but for psychological reasons, or often simply on the side. The question then is: Why am I eating when my body is not hungry? Out of boredom or loneliness, out of routine, frustration, or stress? Am I trying to feed my soul? The next step is to eliminate the reasons for this newly identified non-hungry eating, and anyone who then eats only when truly hungry instead of emotionally eating will surely lose some unnecessary kilos on their own. For many, this "pathological soul-feeding" is not so easy to shake off—in that case, professional psychological help is recommended to banish non-hungry eating from your life. Because this compensatory food intake, used to temporarily numb and swallow negative feelings, is a major problem in obesity. As early as 2011, the University of California was able to show in a study (Daubenmier et al. 2011) that greater mindfulness of bodily signals such as hunger, satiety, and pleasure helps to lose excess weight in the long term. Without special diets. It is also essential not to impose strict bans on favorite foods such as chocolate, cake, or burgers with fries, because the resulting uncontrollable cravings and binge eating quickly ruin weight loss success. With IE, everything is allowed. That's another reason why.

17.7 Losing Weight by Trusting Your Hunger?

Researchers from Florence already provided relevant findings in February 2010: Overweight individuals who eat only when they feel real hunger can lose weight in the long term. By training their true sense of hunger, they continued to lose weight steadily even several years after the study. "Instead of undergoing a diet with uncertain chances of success, training your own sense of hunger could be a key to sustainable weight loss in the future," was the study's conclusion according to the independent aid infodienst from Bonn (aid 2011).—That organization no longer exists; it is now called BZfE, and you know its current opinion on IE. This is also supported by research from US psychologists, who found that naturally slim people almost always eat only when they are truly hungry. And Professor Susanne Klaus from the German Institute of Human Nutrition advised ten years ago to ask yourself before eating: "Am I really hungry right now?" Only those who can honestly answer "yes" to this question should eat (Focus 2011)—and can thus also follow the psychologists' recommendation: "Learn to enjoy the feeling of hunger as a sign of life." This enjoyment should never be neglected, because eating to satisfy hunger is pleasure for the sake of sustaining life. It is less important what you eat, but rather that you experience a deeply fulfilling sense of genuine self-love while eating, through the natural harmony of body, mind, and soul—and, most importantly, that real, biological hunger is and remains your body's primary guide to eating.

17.8 Are You Familiar with This? Interoception!

Because only with this instinctive primal drive as a navigator do we nourish our bodies as they need. And only with real hunger do you sense and enjoy how delicious a truly good meal really tastes. And not only that, because this chapter has a different focus: "It is advisable to learn to pay more attention to your own bodily signals of hunger and satiety and to let your eating behavior be guided by them. If a healthy and normal-weight person, who up to now has had no problems sensing and interpreting interoceptive signals, gains weight after the holidays and Christmas season because they have eaten too much, then that is not too serious." (Hahn 2019)

It can be expected that their eating behavior and weight will relatively easily return to their previously undisturbed eating habits and thus to their usual weight. These people usually do not have pronounced problems perceiving their bodily feedback, nor with self-regulating their behavior, explained Prof. Beate M. Herbert, psychologist, Professor of Biological Psychology & Clinical Psychology at Hochschule Fresenius in Munich and private lecturer at Eberhard Karls University Tübingen, in February 2019 on the science blog "Giving More Attention to Feedback from the Body" of Hochschule Fresenius (Hahn 2019).

What was that technical term again? Interoception. It is the perception and processing of internal bodily signals and their relevance for bodily self-experience. The focus here is on the human ability to perceive signals such as feelings of hunger or satiety. In this sense: Intensify your interoception!

17.9 Hunger—No Stranger

One more little tidbit as a digestif: In 2014, the analysis of a three-country online survey in Germany, Austria, and Switzerland with nearly 2,700 participants found that 61% of people are familiar with their true, physical hunger (Knop 2014). This result confirms a representative survey by the Society for Consumer Research (GfK) from 2012, in which 76% of respondents stated that they recognize their real hunger (Kolb 2012). Both surveys, by the way, contradict the assumption of all total deniers of intuitive eating who claim that people have lost touch with their sense of hunger.

17.10 Hara Hachi bu—Not Related to Hui Buh

To conclude this chapter, let's take another look far to the East: Closely related to IE is the Asian eating wisdom known as "Hara hachi bu" (Hhb). This Japanese saying originally comes from the island of Okinawa, where people live in a "Blue Zone," meaning they have particularly long lifespans. Hara hachi bu: While it may sound like a relative of the castle ghost Hui Buh, it actually means "fill your stomach only to 80%." Hhb is a special form of mindful eating, where one must pay attention to the body's signals—because you start listening to your body again and learn to sense when your stomach has had enough food. At its core, you intuitively learn not to eat beyond the point of satiety. As with IE, no specific foods are forbidden. All of this is intended not only to prevent overweight, but also to reduce the risk of numerous diseases and to extend life overall—there is, as usual, no causal evidence for these promises, but more mindfulness and attention to your own body will certainly do no harm, quite the opposite—whether IE or Hhb or whatever this most natural form of eating is called elsewhere in the world… it can be your real alternative to hypocaloric diets to achieve your biological feel-good weight.

17.11 No Fear of Your Own Self

If you still have some doubts about your own intuitive eating ability, let me leave you with a few motivating lines from *Spiegel online* for your culinary heart: "If I only eat what I feel like, I'll be eating chocolate all the time! Many people fear that they will eat too much, too fatty, or too sweet if they don't control themselves. But is that really the case? Not necessarily. Nutrition scientists now believe that, in the long run, people eat more balanced and relaxed when they listen to their gut feeling. However, this means that you really do have to pay attention to your own body and its signals. Those who more often ask themselves questions like 'What is good for me?' or 'How hungry am I right now?' gradually develop a good personal nutrition compass." (Otto 2020)

In this spirit: Culinary navigation with your own intuitive nutrition compass! The info box "IE compact" below provides you with the essential basic "tools" for this.

17.12 Intuition Meets Ethics—Ethuition

Intuitive eating is the biological path to the most natural human diet. But nowadays, this purely physical level is only one of the two fundamental decision-making bases of personal relevance. Intuitive eating alone is no longer enough for many on the way to the "culinary paradise of complete satisfaction"—it has to be more. Why? You'll find out in the following brief excursus on "holistic eating."

Good, healthy, and right: Eating has become a highly emotional topic, one in which nowadays everyone seems to want to have a say. Whereas in the past, positive emotions such as enjoyment, pleasure, sensuality, and delight were primarily associated with pleasant thoughts of food, today's reality is often quite different: Morality, ideological beliefs, animal welfare or nature conservation, and health ideals "sit at the table" and engage in heated debate (in one's own head). All of this puts people under increasing personal and social pressure when it comes to nutrition: "Goodbye, lightheartedness"—for many, their own diet has become a stressful hot-button issue, and it's especially annoying when it comes to *"healthy"* eating.

Yesterday, fats were the villains, today carbohydrates are unhealthy—and tomorrow, perhaps proteins will be in the dock. In addition to countless "toothless" observational studies, overwhelming masses of official rules and recommendations, and the myriads of self-proclaimed experts, coaches, and influencers, actors, singers, dancers, and unqualified celebrities are also writing all sorts of books about how they have finally discovered the "holy grail of healthy eating"—and, of course, they want to share this enlightenment with the whole world, preferably via social media. And as if all that weren't enough, culinary happiness is further "completed" by a host of "better-eater hypes," each claiming to have found the one true path to "eternal health and slimness"—and, of course, exclusively so, by always leaving something out: low carb, keto, vegan, paleo. Intermittent fasting and clean eating are just some of the top topics among eating hypes—all, of course, combinable à la carte for the ultimate, perfectly healthy eating happiness. Amidst this ever-growing info-overload, many are now faced with the culinary question of all questions:

Who should you believe, who is right, what is fact, what is fake—what can, should, and may I still eat with a clear conscience?

The answer is quite simple: Ignore the entire aforementioned "crazy-making faction" and trust only yourself when it comes to eating—and do so doubly!

In the past 20 years, not only have thousands of nutrition studies been published—rules and trends as well as experts and "nutrition gurus" also come and go. At the end of the hypes, instead of the realization "Now I finally know what healthy eating is!" there is always only one thing left: the same old unanswered questions, paired with new uncertainty, which is immediately replaced by the next "generation of nutrition wisdom and the books of its apostles"—and which, instead of leading to the promised land of eating, once again leads to sobering nothingness. It's always the same pattern, repeating every few years. The reason is simple: Nutrition science is a pitiable branch of science that, due to its massive limitations, cannot provide proof (causal evidence), but only correlations (statistical associations)—and on that basis, at best, hypotheses and assumptions can be generated, but certainly no recommendations. No healthy person needs nutritional science, and even less the made-up rules of institutions, gurus, popes, coaches, and influencers.

Intentions: Power and Interpretive Authority—or Money

That is why, year after year, "new pigs of healthy eating" are driven through the village. The respective pig drivers have two motivations: Either they want to retain power and interpretive authority, or it's about money: making a quick buck with short-lived nutrition hypes. All of this comes and goes at such a rapid pace because the plain truth is this: There is absolutely no proof of healthy eating! So the reverse question arises: Who knows best what healthy eating should be, if science cannot provide this knowledge? Quite simply, there can only be one: And that is your own body—only by fully trusting your own body can you find the path to an absolutely individual healthy diet that provides your body with all the nutrients it needs to live. Ergo, the credo is:

There are as many healthy diets as there are people, because every person eats differently.

This level of bodily trust is called **INTUITION.** Intuitive eating (IE) is the most natural, (bio)logical, and best form of human nutrition, because only it can recognize and fulfill the unique needs of your own body. IE is the basis, the foundation of the right, personally perfectly fitting diet. When am I truly hungry, what do I crave, what tastes good to me, when am I full, and above all: What do I tolerate well, what can my stomach and intestines digest effortlessly? These are the core questions and "guardrails" of IE.

Now you may be thinking: "Well, wonderful, then I'll just eat what makes me feel good physically, what does me good, and the topic of 'healthy eating' is basically settled!" That is, from a purely physical-physiological perspective, absolutely correct—but it's one-dimensional and therefore too short-sighted. Because the aforementioned **"double"** trust in yourself when it comes to eating has, in addition to intuition, a second, equally relevant level that, especially nowadays, also needs to be satisfied:

Also listen to your personal **ETHICS.** This level of trust in your mind, your attitude, and your personally important "values of life" is the perfect complement to your intuition, allowing you to rationally and thus holistically complete the physical part, your feelings—like Yin & Yang. Your personal compass of values becomes the guide for your intuition.

Only by combining these two levels will you find the best diet for yourself—the one that makes you completely happy and satisfied. Because on the one hand: If you listen only to your body, you quickly slide into an "ethical dilemma." The mind, a guilty conscience, garnished with shame, gnaws at you: "Am I buying correctly, am I supporting the right people, is my money as a consumer going where I want it to?" On the other hand: If I buy and eat food primarily rationally, that is, purely guided by reason, based on my personal value standards, without giving the intuitive level equal consideration, then this "rational bias" can lead to physical and psychological problems, perhaps to eating disorders and illnesses.

Therefore, the key to your best eating lies in the symbiosis of both levels:

Harmonize body & mind
Combine health & enjoyment
Merge ethics & intuition

The combination of both is: Follow your **ETHUITION**—that's how simple it is to eat right in harmony with yourself. You don't need anything more, honestly. Nutrition based on your doubly unique Ethuition gives you security, confidence, and the steadfast knowledge that you are doing the right thing—holistically, because your two most important and personal decision-making levels are now resonating in harmonious unison.

Goodbye self-doubt, welcome *clarity*.
Ciao discomfort, hello *contentment*.
Bye insecurity, hi *self-confidence*.
Bye mental merry-go-round, hello *lightness*.

Current societal developments show a new understanding of **"nutrition on a larger scale,"** which merges the well-being of the environment and society with individual well-being. And that is exactly what many people are looking for—because they want to end the endless brooding over the supposedly right diet. The way to achieve this: From now on, let your Ethuition make quick, clear, and "unassailable" decisions that (not only) do you real good and give you the relaxing feeling of steadfast self-confidence: "Very nice, everything done right!"

Are you interested in actually experiencing this wonderful emotion? Then I recommend my new foundational book (2024, KDP [Kindle-Direct-Publishing]), which is dedicated exclusively and very specifically to this essential area of life: **"FINALLY EATING RIGHT—Enjoying honestly with a clear conscience—Trust your ETHICS & INTUITION"**

In the book, you will first learn, based on current studies, all the relevant basics of why science can provide neither proof of healthy nutrition nor of unhealthy foods. On this foundation of "culinary catharsis" (clearing your mind), your further knowledge of intuitive eating, the core ethical questions, and the symbiosis of both—Ethuition—can then flourish undisturbed, so that with each new day you gradually develop a "native flow" and continue to grow.

Perhaps an unshakable trust in the power of your intuition and the strength of your ethics will grow within you. In any case, just as a precaution: Have fun merging both levels and entering your new era of nutrition.

Info box: "IE Compact—Your New Eating Class"

IE offers new **freedom in eating**, because IE makes you

- free from eating stress, health food terror, and dietary constraints
- free from external control
- able to make your own eating decisions again—because only you decide

The "IE quick guide" in 3 steps:

- *Step 1*: Don't believe nutrition myths—neither those of the better-eating gurus, influencers, and health food popes nor the "rules of healthy eating."
- *Step 2:* Recognize your own essential feelings: hunger, desire, enjoyment, satiety, tolerance, and the "groan from deep in your belly."
- *Step 3:* Notice the difference between emotional eating and real hunger. Strengthen your self-awareness.

The following 11 practical everyday tips will help you eat mindfully and intuitively:

1. Only eat when you are hungry. Don't be afraid to let your hunger build up a bit. The stronger the hunger, the better the food you truly like will taste. There are no right or wrong times to eat.
2. Eat only what you crave and what tastes good to you.
3. Tune in mindfully to your body: Notice good tolerance and digestibility (the be-all and end-all of IE) and pay attention to it.
4. Give yourself time (especially at the beginning), be patient with yourself.
5. Don't weigh anything or look up calories in tables.
6. Learn to feel (truly pleasantly) full again. So eat enough until you are full—and not constantly too little (because that will "breed" cravings!).
7. Accept your natural weight (= biological feel-good weight).
8. Don't let yourself get too distracted, focus on what you are doing: eating with enjoyment. And: Slow down!
9. No foods are forbidden. Everything is allowed. There are no healthy or unhealthy, good or bad foods.
10. Inspire yourself with unfamiliar delights/always try new things, explore the full spectrum of available foods. Get to know the entire range of flavors of natural foods.
11. Experience food with all your senses: smell, taste, touch, feel. Also, when preparing and cooking: The more initiative you take, the more "connection" is created between you and your meal.

The Most Important Points of the Chapter

If you do not want to go on a diet but instead trust intuitive eating as your preferred way of eating, the following applies: Eat only when you experience true, physical hunger, and only eat what you genuinely crave, what tastes really delicious to you, and what you tolerate well—trust your intuitive body navigator, which guides you with its feelings while eating. If you also learn to recognize when you are truly full, then you have found the key to your individual, physically and biologically optimal desired and feel-good weight.

References

aid (2011) Bauchgefühl statt Diät: Wer sein Hungergefühl schult, kann langfristig abnehmen. https://pressreleasemag.de/2010/02/bauchgefuehl-statt-diaet-wer-sein-hungergefuehl-schult-kann-langfristig-abnehmen/. Accessed 6. Sept. 2020

Artiles et al (2019) Mindful eating and common diet programs lower body weight similarly: systematic review and meta-analysis. Obesitx Rev. https://doi.org/10.1111/obr.12918

Daubenmier et al (2011) Mindfulness intervention for stress eating to reduce cortisol and abdominal fat among overweight and obese women: an exploratory randomized controlled study. J Obesity. https://doi.org/10.1155/2011/651936

Focus (2011) Abnehmen mit einfachen Tricks: auf den Körper hören. https://www.focus.de/gesundheit/ernaehrung/abnehmen/tid-20542/abnehmen-schlank-ohne-hungern-auf-den-koerper-hoeren_aid:575277.html. Accessed 6. Sept. 2020

Freitag-Ziegler G (2019) Intuitiv essen oder nach Ernährungsregeln? https://www.bzfe.de/inhalt/intuitiv-essen-oder-nach-ernaehrungsregeln-34862.html. Accessed 6. Sept. 2020

gesund.bund (2020) Wie sieht eine gesunde Ernährung aus? https://gesund.bund.de/gesunde-ernaehrung. Accessed 6. Sept. 2020

Hahn M (2019) Fastenzeit: „Rückmeldungen aus dem Körper mehr Gehör schenken“. https://www.adhibeo.de/fastenzeit-rueckmeldungen-aus-dem-koerper-mehr-gehoer-schenken/. Accessed 6. Sept. 2020

Knop U (2014) Aktuelle Umfrage: 61% kennen ihr Hungergefühl. https://www.echte-esser.de/echter-hunger-statt-xter-diaet-der-schluessel-zum-wunschgewicht.html. Accessed 6. Sept. 2020

Kolb A (2012) Echter Hunger (GfK-Umfrage). https://www.echte-esser.de/tl_files/files/GfK_Hunger_repraesentativ_Feb-12.pdf. Accessed 6. Sept. 2020

Lück I (2019) Einfach aufs Bauchgefühl hören. https://landeszentrum-bw.de/,Lde/wissen/Ernaehrungsinformation/Ernaehrungswissen/Intuitive+Ernaehrung. Accessed 6. Sept. 2020

Müller C (2019) Warum ist es (nicht) so schwierig, sich ausgewogen zu ernähren? https://www.bzfe.de/inhalt/ernaehrungswissen-616.html. Accessed 6. Sept. 2020

Otto A (2020) Körper, hör die Signale! https://www.spiegel.de/gesundheit/ernaehrung/koerper-hoer-die-signale-a-d8bca75b-6ebf-4376-88f7-cbd97d10feb3. Accessed 6. Sept. 2020

18

Is there a "Shortcut" to Your Desired Weight?

At the very end of the book, we address an "additional question" that is repeatedly asked in the context of the long-term life project "becoming and staying slim"—namely: Can I shortcut the path to my desired weight? Are there agents or active substances that can accelerate or facilitate weight loss?

Many people would certainly like the answer to be a "turbo fat-melting pill" or a "kilo-elimination injection" that makes unwanted body fat disappear as if by "magic"… Up until 2023, we would have quickly burst this daydream bubble: "Forget it," would have been the answer. But since then, the "world of weight loss" has changed:

Because since 2023, two "weight loss injections" have been approved as medications in Germany—which are being discussed as "game changers" in the fight against overweight.

So that you, too, can better assess and evaluate these pharmaceutical agents—and decide whether and how they might fit into your own "path to your desired weight"—you will find below all the essential information on the substances currently available (as of May 2025):

First, in 2023, the weight loss injection **"Wegovy"** (active ingredient: semaglutide) came onto the market—it has since become very

U. Knop, *Successful and Sustainable Weight Loss*,
https://doi.org/10.1007/978-3-662-72477-4_18

well known, allegedly because many celebrities such as Elon Musk and Robbie Williams use the drug to lose weight (at least, that's what they claim publicly). This substance is approved for adults with a body mass index (BMI) of 30 or higher (obesity) as well as for those who are "overweight" but not quite as severely (BMI of 27 or higher), provided they also suffer from certain comorbidities. The second weight loss injection is called **"Mounjaro"** (active ingredient: tirzepatide)—it is also approved for the aforementioned indications.

Both active substances are not new—they have been used for many years to treat type 2 diabetes ("diabetes mellitus")—and since 2023, they can now also be specifically prescribed for overweight or obese individuals who do not have diabetes.

It is important to note that all users not only have to inject themselves, but also absolutely must change their diet and increase their physical activity.

Both injections can only be prescribed by a doctor with a prescription—but patients must pay the costs themselves, as health insurance does not cover these "lifestyle medications." And it's not cheap: a month's supply costs several hundred euros.

The Mechanism of Action of Weight Loss Injections

Tirzepatide and semaglutide belong to the class of active substances known as "GLP-1 receptor agonists" (also called GLP-1 analogues, i.e., GLP-1 "copies"), meaning they mimic the action of the body's own gut hormone GLP-1, which is released when we eat. Its effects include, on the one hand, increasing insulin secretion from the pancreas, which can lower blood sugar levels more precisely than other medications—hence their previous use in diabetes. On the other hand, it affects the satiety center in our brain, as it reduces hunger and appetite and leads to slower gastric emptying and longer satiety. Overall, those using the "weight loss injections" feel less hungry, are fuller, and therefore eat less.

An amusing anecdote: The story of weight loss injections is similar to that of Viagra (active ingredient: sildenafil), which was originally developed as a heart medication, but whose side effect—"stable erection"—turned out to be much more lucrative! The same is true here: the (desired) side effect of "weight loss" is much more interesting, and thus more profitable, than the main effect of "lowering and controlling blood sugar."

How Effective are Tirzepatide and Semaglutide for Weight Loss?
A **study** in the renowned medical journal *JAMA* examined "Semaglutide vs. Tirzepatide for Weight Loss in Adults with Overweight or Obesity" (Rodriguez 2024). In this comparative study, the researchers were able to show that tirzepatide led to significantly greater weight loss than semaglutide—while the side effects of both substances were comparable.

A weight loss of more than 10% within one year was achieved by 62% of tirzepatide patients and 38% of the semaglutide group. **Even more than 15% weight loss was achieved** by 42% of the T-patients and 18% of the S-group.

The "big but": More than half of the participants dropped out of the study—and thus the therapy! The dropout rate was similar in both groups. The reasons for discontinuation were not surveyed—but it is likely due in particular to the high costs of this self-pay therapy or the known side effects.

Pharmaceutical Law: No Effect Without Side Effects
Above all, "gastrointestinal" side effects occur, i.e., in the digestive tract: nausea, vomiting, abdominal pain, as well as a feeling of fullness and loss of appetite. It is already being speculated that these unwanted side effects alone may contribute to some of the weight loss; simply because those who experience severe gastrointestinal problems eat much less (can and want to) and thus automatically lose weight. In principle, the following applies: Since the active substances are administered at significantly higher doses than in the "pure" diabetes injections, the side effects—and thus the weight loss triggered by them—could also be more pronounced.

Another aesthetic side effect that visibly counteracts the "quickly becoming slimmer and more beautiful" is the so-called Wegovy face. This refers to a sagging, drooping face that results from the fact that, due to the sometimes very rapid weight reduction, tightening (fat) tissue in the face is also lost. As a result, those who slim down quickly with injections develop this disadvantageously sunken and older-looking facial structure, plus a haggard facial expression caused by the rapid loss of volume.

Last but not least, discontinuing the injections leads to the yo-yo effect—that is, the lost kilos quickly return, and weight increases significantly again without the injections. Therefore, the high dropout rate in the aforementioned recent study of over 50% is very concerning. Because, in fact, the active substances must be used for life to maintain the effect—while currently neither long-term risks nor data on achieving important goals ("clinical endpoints") such as fewer heart attacks, strokes, or cancer are known. Put simply: The first "weight loss injectors are the guinea pigs in the wild."

Large-Scale Study Shows Broad Spectrum of Effects

Of interest in this context is a large-scale study from 2025, in which glucagon-like peptide-1 receptor agonists (GLP-1-RA) were systematically investigated for the first time with regard to various effects on 175 (!) health problems and diseases (Xie 2025). The researchers found that the weight loss injections not only lower blood sugar and weight—but also change the risks for various complaints and diseases in users. The authors report that GLP-1-RA can have not only numerous positive additional effects, but also some negative risks.

Therefore, it is important that all doctors who prescribe weight loss injections inform each individual patient in detail about their personal risks.

You also have to be prepared to inject yourself once a week, probably for life—and not everyone is willing or able to do that. Ultimately, the decision for or against weight loss injections will always be made by the doctor on a case-by-case basis, after an individual benefit-risk assessment has been carried out.

Key Question: Do Weight Loss Injections Work all by Themselves?

The dream of "just get an injection and lose weight effortlessly" will not come true—because without a long-term, individually tailored change in diet and sufficient physical activity, you will not remain slim in the long run. As soon as you stop the injections and do nothing else, you will quickly regain a significant amount of weight—the yo-yo effect is inevitable. And who wants to inject themselves with weight loss medication every week for the rest of their life and pay thousands of euros per year for it? At present, no one knows how long-term injections will affect weight, for example, whether the weight-reducing effect will eventually wear off, whether new, stronger side effects will emerge, and how potential "injection dependency" might impact mental health and thus the development of eating disorders.

All in all, much remains unclear in this regard. At the moment, the injections are only sensible as a supplement and support to a comprehensive obesity therapy—but the **individual, permanent lifestyle change** remains essential, because without it, nothing will work in the long term except for the number on the scale to quickly rise again.

Key Points of the Chapter

- My recommendation: For your "ideal weight project," rely first and foremost on yourself and your own initiative—and steer clear of weight loss injections. If you absolutely need pharmaceutical assistance because you cannot manage on your own, then discuss all the opportunities and, above all, the risks of weight loss injections openly with your doctor—and only decide which path to take after a few days of consideration. As a general and very important piece of advice: Stay away from over-the-counter dietary supplements (DS) from the internet. They promise the world but deliver nothing. By law, DS are not allowed to have any effect; legally, they are only considered food. Lack of efficacy is the least of your worries—depending on what is mixed in, internet DS can also be hazardous to your health.

References

Rodriguez et al (2024) Semaglutide vs Tirzepatide for Weight Loss in Adults With Overweight or Obesity. https://doi.org/10.1001/jamainternmed.2024.2525

Xie et al (2025) Mapping the effectiveness and risks of GLP-1 receptor agonists. Nat Med (2025). https://doi.org/10.1038/s41591-024-03412-w

will quickly regain a significant amount of weight—the yo-yo effect is inevitable. And who wants to inject themselves with weight loss medication every week for the rest of their life and pay thousands of euros per year for it? At present, no one knows how long-term injections will affect weight, for example, whether the weight-reducing effect will eventually wear off, whether new, stronger side effects will emerge, and how potential "injection dependency" might impact mental health and thus the development of eating disorders.

All in all, much remains unclear in this regard. At the moment, the injections are only sensible as a supplement and support to a comprehensive obesity therapy—but the **individual, permanent lifestyle change** remains essential, because without it, nothing will work in the long term except for the number on the scale to quickly rise again.

Key Points of the Chapter

- My recommendation: For your "ideal weight project," rely first and foremost on yourself and your own initiative—and steer clear of weight loss injections. If you absolutely need pharmaceutical assistance because you cannot manage on your own, then discuss all the opportunities and, above all, the risks of weight loss injections openly with your doctor—and only decide which path to take after a few days of consideration. As a general and very important piece of advice: Stay away from over-the-counter dietary supplements (DS) from the internet. They promise the world but deliver nothing. By law, DS are not allowed to have any effect; legally, they are only considered food. Lack of efficacy is the least of your worries—depending on what is mixed in, internet DS can also be hazardous to your health.

References

Rodriguez et al (2024) Semaglutide vs Tirzepatide for Weight Loss in Adults With Overweight or Obesity. https://doi.org/10.1001/jamainternmed.2024.2525

Xie et al (2025) Mapping the effectiveness and risks of GLP-1 receptor agonists. Nat Med (2025). https://doi.org/10.1038/s41591-024-03412-w

19

Afterword: Dear Women, Dear Men ...

To conclude your project "Losing Weight/Achieving Your Desired Weight," I would like to give you one key takeaway. My message to all of you out there who are aiming for a long-term change in diet and thus (often visibly) reshaping your body is short and clear:

Your body belongs to you. It is your unique organism, and you should love it completely—because you only have this one. So remember: Don't let self-proclaimed nutrition gurus, weight-loss experts, or diet authorities tell you what you should eat or how you should lose weight. Only you, in the holistic harmony of body, soul, and mind, truly know how to shape your body into one you love and with which you love to live. For life. In this spirit:

Be yourself. Be authentic.

Important Note

This book and its guidance for individual, sustainable weight reduction are intended for psychosomatically **healthy** individuals who do not suffer from mental or physical illnesses, organic dysfunctions, or metabolic disorders. Implementation of the recommendations is at your own risk and

U. Knop, *Successful and Sustainable Weight Loss*,
https://doi.org/10.1007/978-3-662-72477-4_19

without any guarantee. The information in this book does not replace professional advice/diagnosis or personal treatment of illnesses by physicians/nutritional medicine specialists. The content is not intended to be used to make disease diagnoses or to initiate therapies independently.